WOMAN

designed
by God

DR
AMANDA HESS

DR
JEREMY HESS

elevate
faith

Cover Design by Arthur Cherry

Interior Layout by Leslie Hertling

Interior Graphics by Bobby Kuber

Published in Boise, Idaho by Elevate Faith, a division of Elevate Publishing. www.elevatepub.com

This book may be purchased in bulk for educational, business, ministry, or promotional use.

For information please email: info@elevatepub.com.

ISBN: 978-1-937498-48-1

Printed in the United States of America

To all the women who seek to understand
a more natural way of living, who cry out
to God for a better way; desire to live a life
full of health, vitality and longevity;
wish to teach other women, their children and
grandchildren natural laws and
holistic methods of living from the inside-out;
pray and plan to reach their God-given destiny
and purpose for their lives.

– Drs. Amanda and Jeremy Hess

Advanced Praise for
Woman Designed by God

Drs. Jeremy and Amanda Hess have done a brilliant job of packaging life-transforming information that can make your life pain-free and much more enjoyable. Who knew things like shampoo and face wash could actually contribute to major illnesses, including cancer? The success stories from everyday people are sure to inspire you to another level of healthy living.

Jillian Chambers
Lead Pastor of Oasis Church, Nashville, TN

Today, women in our society are faced with many health and beauty standards based on what they see on television or in a magazine. *Woman Designed by God* is a breath of fresh air detailing how to be a healthy, natural, and beautiful woman. This will be a go-to guide for years to come for women of all ages looking to live life naturally, the way God designed.

Dr. Samantha Brown
Specific, Scientific Chiropractor
Bright Life Chiropractic

Woman Designed by God is an easy to read, straightforward tool for educating women in our pharmaceutical-crazed culture.
Sherri Dodd
Founder and CEO, Advance Global Coaching

I have found this book to be of great inspiration and believe that it will also greatly impact the lives of those who read it. Drs. Jeremy and Amanda Hess have great understanding of God's word and how He created the body, as well how the body functions. Their knowledge is cemented in this book. Truly, when someone shares what God has placed in their hearts, something beautiful happens, and that is the case here.

Evangelist Martha Ekua Harley
Founder and CEO, Amazing Grace Evangelical International Ministries, Inc.

Doctors Jeremy and Amanda Hess have created a comprehensive guide to a woman's health that is both inspiring and transformational. The principles they share are timeless. This book is shockingly eye-opening and will change the way you think about your health, and if taken to heart, could enhance, prolong or even save your life.

Pastor Charla Turner
Turning Point Church
McDonough, GA

In *Woman Designed by God*, Drs. Jeremy and Amanda Hess brilliantly combine biblical principles with practical solutions for improving your health and the health of the entire family. This book is fascinating and an easy read. I plan to share it with all my patients.

Meri Warbrick
ND,CCT,CLT

My entire life is my spiritual life, and taking care of my health is worship; our bodies are temples. Thank you, Drs. Amanda and Jeremy, for teaching us how to live powerfully.

Pam Kennard
Nspire Outreach

The creation of woman was one of God's crowning achievements. *Woman Designed by God* highlights the benefits of embracing how God designed a woman's body. It reminds women that each part of her body serves a purpose and encourages women to research natural methods to promote healing and well-being.

Charity Haulk
Founder of Fruit of the Womb—
Birth Naturally, Live Naturally.
www.fruitofthewomb.info

It has been exciting to see the Hesses' journey into capturing the heart of providing a healthy home and life, all through a book. They have worked very diligently to give women some of the steps to living a whole life. I wish I had been given some of the same encouragements and directives when I started my path into a healthy lifestyle, and I wait in expectation of the national success of this book and how it impacts communities to move in such lifestyles. Women need to be encouraged to guide their families and themselves—and this book does just that!

Tanya J. Trail
CPM - Midwife
www.LaboringHands.com

table of contents

Chapter 1 Questioning a Hidden Health Crisis | 1

Chapter 2 Cover Girl | 9

Chapter 3 Tickled Pink for Men in White | 27

Chapter 4 Body Built for a Baby | 41

Chapter 5 Woman's Oath of Health | 63

Chapter 6 Sweet Curves | 81

Chapter 7 That Time of the Month | 95

Chapter 8 Just Like Mom | 111

Chapter 9 Natural Living: Designed by God | 131

1.

Questioning a Hidden Health Crisis

How many of you think you could have taken better care of your health or done things differently over the past 10 years? How many of you think that you or someone you know is taking too many pharmaceuticals? Raise your hand if you know a child on constant pharmaceuticals for ear infections, asthma, or attention deficit disorder. Raise your hand if you believe that this next generation, either your children or your grandchildren, just seem to be sicker than previous generations. These are the kinds of questions that we ask folks that come in and out of our chiropractic practice each week, and it never fails that hands fly up in response.

Every day, we hear sentences such as, "I wish I would have known; I would have done things differently," or, "The doctor never told me that was even an option." These are the unfortunate clichés we hear so often from practice members. As we teach how God designed the body in His perfect image, whole, healthy and full of vitality, we have to ask: Why does health have to be so complicated in our current culture? We live in the United States of America, where we have supposedly the best healthcare available. We consume more pharmaceuticals than any other country in the world. In 2012, North America accounted for 41 percent of world pharmaceutical sales. In fact, according to IMS (Intercontinental Marketing Services) data, 62 percent of sales of new pharmaceutical drugs launched from 2007 to 2011 were on the U.S. market (as opposed to only 18 percent on the European market).[1] The United States spends more money on healthcare costs than any other country in the world, which should translate to us being first in overall health in the world. Sadly, however, that is not the case in so many areas of our health, when comparing statistics of life expectancy, maternal mortality or infant mortality, just to name a few.

We find that countless women have a sheer lack of knowledge on many of the subjects that we will address in this book. That's why we believe in reaching out to women and showing them that there is a better way, that our bodies were designed to function and heal from the inside out, and that we were truly designed by God with a uniqueness about us that totally separates us from our male counterparts! Many attributes of this feminine singularity will be written about and shared in *Woman Designed by God*.

The healthcare industry's attitude toward women raises many thought-provoking questions. Should we really believe that in our teen years, we need pharmaceuticals for acne, and our menstrual cycle should be our nemesis? Is it totally safe for us and all of our twenty-something girlfriends to take birth control pills for many years? Why are so many of us and our "healthy-looking" friends having fertility issues? And for those

1. "The Pharmaceutical Industry in Figures." European Federation of Pharmaceutical Industries and Associations. http://www.efpia.eu/uploads/Figures_Key_Data_2013.pdf, 4.

U.S. Healthcare

Overall Quality & Expenses

COUNTRY RANKINGS	AUS	CAN	FRA	GER	NETH	NZ	NOR	SWE	SWIZ	UK	US
Top 2* / Middle / Bottom 2*											
OVERALL RANKING (2013)	4	10	9	5	5	7	7	3	2	1	11
Quality Care	2	9	8	7	5	4	11	10	3	1	5
Effective Care	4	7	9	6	5	2	11	10	8	1	3
Safe Care	3	10	2	6	7	9	11	5	4	1	7
Coordinated Care	4	8	9	10	5	2	7	11	3	1	6
Patient-Centered Care	5	8	10	7	3	6	11	9	2	1	4
Access	8	9	11	2	4	7	6	4	2	1	9
Cost-Related Problem	9	5	10	4	8	6	3	1	7	1	11
Timeliness of Care	6	11	10	4	2	7	8	9	1	3	5
Efficiency	4	10	8	9	7	3	4	2	6	1	11
Equity	5	9	7	4	8	10	6	1	2	2	11
Healthy Lives	4	8	1	7	5	9	6	2	3	10	11
Health Expenditures /Capita, 2011**	$3,800	$4,522	$4,118	$4,495	$5,099	$3,182	$5,669	$3,925	$5,643	$3,405	$8,508

U.S. ranked dead last in **overall healthcare** according to the CommonWealth Fund.

U.S. ranked **most expensive healthcare system** according to the Common-Wealth Fund.

Notes: *Includes ties. ** Expenditures in $US PPP (purchasing power parity); Australian $ data are from 2010. Source: Calculated by the Commonwealth Fund based on 2011 International Health Policy Survey of Sicker Adults; 2012 International Health Policy Survey of Primary Care Physicians; 2013 International Health Policy Survey; Commonwealth Fund *National Scorecard 2011*; World Health Organization; and Organization for Economic Cooperation and Development, OECD Health Data, *2013* (Paris: OECD, Nov. 2013).

who are having children, why is it that 1 out of 3 women has a cesarean section surgery? Why is it no longer standard procedure for a woman to have a natural, uncomplicated, un-medicated birth? Is it normal for 1 out of 4 women to be taking anti-depressants? Will it be more profitable for the pharmaceutical industry to actually find a cure for cancer? Why does it seem that everybody we know eventually has been prescribed blood pressure and cholesterol medication? And why, all of a sudden, do we see these amazing Alzheimer's care facilities being built nowadays?

Are we the only ones asking these questions? Are we the only people that believe women—and the public at large—need to be more educated about their health and healthcare decisions? Our bodies are our temples. It is our responsibility to take care of our temple. Did God design us to be dependent on Him and His design, or to be dependent on pharmaceutical drugs and surgeries on a mainstream basis (not an emergency basis), popping pills everyday with the false belief system that these pills will keep us healthy?

Why don't we trust in our body's perfect design and ability to heal itself? The "why" lies in our beliefs that we always need to suppress symptoms or cover up the problem. In our minds, it makes perfect sense! If we have a blemish on our face, we use makeup to cover it up. If we have a digestive issue or a migraine, it would seem logical to use a drug to suppress and cover up the symptom. If we have heavy, uncontrollable bleeding or uterine tumors, cut them out

> Our bodies are our temples. It is our responsibility to take care of our temple.

or get a hysterectomy. Whatever part of our body that is not functioning normally, we will use a pharmaceutical for as long as possible to suppress the symptom and to delay the need for surgery.

This mentality begins when we are children. Most of us grew up using a medicine cabinet, with our parents and doctors teaching us to treat ailments with pills until surgery becomes the only option. Comically, this approach seems almost like fixing a car. The only difference is that your car is a machine, with parts that break. Your car is not a living, breathing, healing creation like your body. In fact, if taken care of properly, your body is not meant to break down, as the current healthcare culture wants you to believe. Sure, traumatic events do occur, but take a moment to compare your heart to a car engine. Your heart beats about 70 times a minute for 80 to 120 years, without ever stopping. Your car engine is not even close—it works maybe 8 to 10 years, if you're lucky. As women, we need to rethink and renew the way we view our bodies. We should not assume that we will ultimately get this disease or that condition because we are aging, or because our mothers and grandmothers passed it down to us.

We believe if we do things the right way, we can live a life full of health, vitality, and longevity the way God created us. He is our Provider, but that doesn't always mean that the provision will come on a silver platter. We have to be educated and guide ourselves to make the right choices. Just like following a recipe to make the perfect dinner dish, the same goes for our bodies and our health. If we follow the recipe and take the steps to think correctly about what we put in and on our bodies, then we can expect to get better results. Now, we will never say this is easy, as our society is set up to lure us into quick fixes, fast food, and immediate gratification. However, the quick-fix mentality typically ends up with long-term health failures. The law of cause and effect plays a big role here, and the consequences for breaking the natural laws of health and healing will ultimately result in dysfunction and disease of the body.

Like many of you, we used to choose the path of least resistance when it concerned our health. As we look back about 15 to 20 years ago, when we really weren't taking care of our bodies, we viewed ourselves as healthy if we looked good and didn't express any symptoms, such as coughing or sneezing. We were exercising to be fit and eating what we thought was an above-average American diet. From the outside looking in, we appeared to be healthy. When a health problem occurred, we would crawl into bed and take whatever was in the medicine cabinet. If it was a crisis, we found ourselves in situations where a doctor was saying we needed to take a drug (which didn't sit well with us) or worse yet, that we needed to schedule a procedure immediately! As we look back now, the problem with our attitude toward health was that we never took the time to question, research or pray about our options, and when in crisis mode, fear always seemed to win out over knowledge. And because we typically knew little about the drug we were going to take, or procedure or surgery that we were signing off on, without realizing it, we were making fear-based decisions out of desperation.

> The power that created your body *can* and *will* heal your body!

We've pondered over the years how we could have done things differently and better, and how we should have made more educated decisions, but we tell ourselves not to live in the past. We know that God has given us a body that can heal itself, even after making poor health decisions or outright abusing our bodies. Just like the renewal of the mind that Paul explains in Romans 12, our bodies are wonderfully and magnificently made and designed by God with a constant renewing of cells, tissue, glands and organs. The power that created your body *can* and *will* heal your body!

As you read this book, we challenge you to renew your vision of health for yourself and your loved ones. Allow yourself to be open to the power of the innate healing potential inside of you that God placed in you when you were conceived and in your mother's womb. When you were birthed into this world, that innate, God-given intelligence didn't leave your body; it's still with you, right now working and functioning in your favor and for your benefit! All you must do is learn to work *with* it, not against it. Examine your current health habits and beliefs and what you can do and/or change to be more committed to your health, so that you may live the healthy life God desires for you. You can not only *be* a Woman Designed by God, but you can *live* like one too!

2.

Cover Girl

You should have seen the look on my husband's face when Alyssa, our 7-year-old daughter, walked into the kitchen with lipstick, eyeshadow, blush, and glitter on her face. It's like his internal *This is not happening!!!* alarm went off, and he blanked out for a moment as Alyssa pranced around the kitchen showing him and her baby brother, Gabriel, how grown-up she looked! With the quick glance I made in his direction to indicate we were just having some girly fun, he calmed down and realized that to Alyssa, it all seemed perfectly innocent...at least for now.

Every girl remembers playing dress up with Mom or a big sister, putting on lipstick or a little eyeshadow for the first time, peering into the mirror and dreaming of being a princess and meeting that prince. It's normal, it's natural, it's what us girls do and what we all did when we were growing up! I remember growing up feeling very awkward about how thin I was. As the "super-skinny disproportioned girl," I clearly remember nicknames such as "Dumbo ears," "Flintstone feet," and "Toothpick legs." So at a young age, I began dancing competitively. For competition day, all the girls would put gobs and gobs of stage makeup on their face and curl their hair with over a hundred small pink rollers. The hair and makeup gave me a new identity. I always felt pretty with my stiff, hairsprayed curls, fake eyelashes, fire-engine-red lipstick, and neon-colored, sequined costumes.

Many women are caught up trying to appear beautiful at all times, going so far as to mask their imperfections. We constantly use products like cosmetics, lotions, soaps, perfumes, hair dye, and the sort! Not only do they make us feel better about ourselves, but also it's what everyone else does.

I remember when my husband, Dr. Jeremy, went to the practice a few years ago off hours to adjust a woman in her 60s who had fallen and was in severe pain. When he got home after taking care of her, he remarked on their conversation. As she was lying on the chiropractic table in agony, she was still so aware of her appearance that she told Dr. Jeremy that he was the second man ever to see her like this. At first, my husband didn't get it. She explained that no man other than her husband had seen her without makeup or hairspray, but today, because she was in such pain, she didn't care that my husband saw her without her being "covered up"!

Throughout adolescence and early adulthood, I never really gave much thought about the safety and/or possible health hazards in any of my cosmetics, hair products, body products, or home products. I also hardly noticed or thought it abnormal when friends were dealing with thyroid issues, chronic migraines, menstrual and fertility problems, or other more serious health concerns at such a young age.

My thinking changed, though, when I started to research what it cost me to look my best. I'm not referring to a monetary cost, but a cost to my overall health and wellbeing. Sure, it can financially cost a bunch to look good and cover up, and doing so is time-consuming in the present, but have you ever wondered if there is a long-term cost of covering up? I believe most women have never given much thought to the subject; I know that for a long time, I didn't ask what (if any) consequences hairsprays, facial cosmetics or other stuff we put on our skin has on our bodies. I didn't question if soaps, lotions, shampoos or deodorants affect you, more than just making you smell good and shine better.

I clearly remember the first (and only) time I had my hair dyed. I had just made the cheerleading team for a local Georgia football team, and we had many sponsors to help us feel and look beautiful on and off the field. We had a chiropractor, massage therapist, a tanning salon, cosmetologists, and free memberships to local dance and fitness clubs. After lining up all 20 of us for makeovers, I was told that they wanted my hair to "pop" more on the field, so I headed to the salon for some auburn colored hair dye. Even though I was a kid who grew up in the 80s, where the popular thing to do was to get a perm in your hair, I always declined fake, chemically-laden permanent curls for no other reason than that I just didn't like them. This time, however, I was at the mercy of beauty professionals. The salon was amazing and for whatever reason I was the lucky girl that the salon owner chose to service. As the dye covered my scalp and hair, I felt tingling sensations and a little burning. I thought, *this is probably normal…no big deal.* I left the salon with my new hair shiny and beautiful. I have to admit that I loved it, and people around me loved it too. They were commenting about how pretty my hair appeared, and all women (including myself) like for others to notice them. The part I didn't love, however, was the itch I felt on my scalp for the next 5 days. It was so bad (an obvious allergic reaction) that I vowed to my husband to never to do it again. After the 5 days of itching, my scalp felt back to normal, and I went on with my regular life activities, ignoring the possibility of any permanent side effects from the hair dye.

Several years went by, and over time, Jeremy and I began to make lifestyle changes in an attempt to live a better and healthier life for the long term. We gradually stopped eating fast food. We began shopping at natural food stores and grocery stores like Whole Foods. I was inquisitive about the different soaps, shampoos, toothpastes, cosmetics and cleaning products sold at these stores. Thus, I began my research. I started to discover new findings, such as one startling study from the UK that found that the average woman exposes her skin to up to 175 different chemicals every day.[1] Most of these chemicals are in the form of makeup and beautification products. Dangerous chemicals—like sulfates, aluminum, parabens, triclosan, petroleum-based products, and various reactive acids—are present in many popular cosmetic products

> The average woman exposes her skin to up to 175 different chemicals every day. Most of these chemicals are in the form of makeup and beautification products.

1. Cochrane, Kira. "Is your beauty regime damaging your health?" *The Guardian.* http://www. theguardian.com/lifeandstyle/2007/sep/11/healthandwellbeing.kiracochrane

today and are absorbed by the skin into the bloodstream. They may also lead to numerous lingering side effects, some of which are thought to have serious repercussions for the user's general health. These chemicals may result in allergic reactions, skin discolorations, headaches, eye infections, depression, thyroid disorders, reproductive issues, breathing problems and possibly even cancer!

At first, like many of you, I had a hard time believing that the FDA and our government regulators would allow these kind of chemicals to be freely used in our cosmetics at such alarming rates. An article from *Natural News* states:

> When it comes to cosmetics and safety, the consumer must keep in mind that there is no U.S. governmental agency regulating products in this category. The FDA can only make recommendations about unsafe chemicals; it is up to the cosmetic companies themselves to do the research into an ingredient's safety or potential dangers. Consumers can draw their own conclusions, but when one looks at Europe and other countries to see what is regulated and compares this list to the list of ingredients on the packages on our drugstore shelves, it is cause for concern. The discrepancy makes it hard to trust the industry. As always, it is up to you, the consumer, to do the research and to become responsible for your own health, in regard to what goes on your body in addition to what goes in it.[2]

2. Sherman, Cathy. "The Dangers in Hair Coloring and Safer Alternatives." *Natural News*. http://www.naturalnews.com/022575_hair_color_chemicals.html#ixzz2seojNWfn.

Another disturbing article I ran across in the early stages of my research examined chemicals called parabens. I discovered that parabens are any of a group of compounds used as preservatives to prevent bacteria, yeast and mold growth in pharmaceuticals, cosmetic products and in the food industry. They have been widely used since the 1950s, and Dr. Arthur Rich, a cosmetic chemist, states that about 85 percent of cosmetics contain these preservatives.[3] Parabens appear in some deodorants and antiperspirants, in addition to personal care products that contain significant amounts of water, such as shampoos, conditioners, lotions, and facial and shower cleansers and scrubs. These parabens, like many other chemicals, ended up being in many of the products I used on a daily basis.

Still, what's the problem? The most disturbing research I initially came across examined the potential relationship between parabens and breast cancer. In the 1990s, parabens were deemed *xenoestrogens*—agents that mimic estrogen in the body. Agents that cause "estrogen disruption" have been linked to breast cancer and reproductive issues. In 2012, the *Journal of Applied Toxicology* found in a study that 99 percent of breast cancer patients had parabens in their breast tissue.[4] Critics of this and other studies argue that noncancerous tissue from healthy breasts wasn't examined to see if parabens were also present there, and that the presence of parabens in tumors doesn't prove that they caused the cancer. However, all this only leads to further concern about the unknown, as many specialists

3. Gage, Eleni. "What Are Parabens—and Do I Need to Worry About Them?" *Real Simple.* http://www.realsimple.com/beauty-fashion/skincare/worry-about-parabens-00000000028428/

4. Barr, L., Metaxas, G., Harbach, C. A. J., Savoy, L. A. and Darbre, P. D. "Measurement of paraben concentrations in human breast tissue at serial locations across the breast from axilla to sternum." *Journal of Applied Toxicology*, 32: 219-232.

Parabens As Preservatives

The Carcinogenic & Estrogenic Dangers

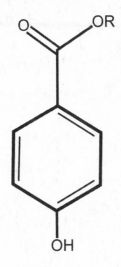

Parabens are used to prevent the growth of microbes in cosmetic products and can be absorbed through skin, blood, and the digestive system. Most commonly used parabens include methylparaben, ethylparaben, propylparaben, butylparaben and heptylparaben.

Parabens mimic estrogen and are known to disrupt hormone function, an effect that may be linked to increased risk of breast cancer and reproductive toxicity.

Parabens can be found in a long laundry list of products, including:

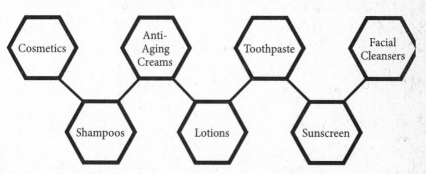

Safe Cosmetics Action Network. "Parabens." Campaign for Safe Cosmetics. http://www.safecosmetics.org/article.php?id=291

will tout there is no clear indicator that parabens are linked to cancer. Both the U.S. Food and Drug Administration and the World Health Organization consider these chemicals safe at low levels. My question is, what about the cumulative effect of countless low-level paraben-containing products used on a daily basis? Obviously, more research needs to be done, but for my family and myself, we choose to use oil-based organic products that don't contain water (which calls for a preservative). You too can find these products, as they will be labeled paraben-free.

As my curiosity continued through the aisles of different health food stores, I noticed that the deodorants were labeled "aluminum-free." I realized that I had no idea what chemicals were in my antiperspirant, nor did it ever cross my mind to think that they may be harmful to my health. The active ingredient in antiperspirants is an aluminum-based compound that temporarily plugs the sweat ducts so that you don't sweat. But many experts believe that by plugging up your sweat ducts, your body cannot purge toxins, which may lead to a cascade effect of chronic toxic overload. Absorption of these chemicals may eventually contribute to cancer and other neurological concerns such as Alzheimer's.

> It doesn't make sense to potentially set the stage for a health crisis in the future, just so I can look and smell good.

Antiperspirants usually are partnered with a deodorant to help you smell good, a combination of other inactive ingredients, and potentially harmful chemicals and the aforementioned parabens. Some recent studies concluded that aluminum-based antiperspirants may increase the risk for breast cancer. The axillary tail (of Spence), the upper-outer quadrant of the breast (i.e. the area nearest to the armpit) is where 50 percent of breast cancer is located, and it's also where we apply antiperspirants every day for many years. Many Internet "experts" have written health articles clearly stating that there is no convincing evidence of these claims, but to be on the safe side until more research has been done, I will buy the natural alternatives and stay aluminum-free. You may see me sweat sometimes, but sweating is a natural, God-given function of the body. It doesn't make sense to purposely inhibit the sweat glands and potentially set the stage for a health crisis in the future, just so I can look and smell good.

As I looked around my house at the ingredients list of common industrial cleaners, shampoos, toothpastes, shaving foam, facial cleansers, body washes, makeup foundations, liquid soaps, laundry detergents and bath products, I found the common ingredients *sodium lauryl sulfate* (SLS), *sodium laureth sulfate* (SLES), *ammonium laurel sulfate* (ALS), and other alias names ending with "sulfate". It seemed like every product listed sulfates as some of the main ingredients, yet when I was shopping in natural food stores, many of the products were labeled "sulfate-free". So what is the purpose of sulfates, and are these sulfates something to be concerned about?

Basically, sulfates are the ingredients that make products lather, foam and bubble. The problem is that they are corrosive cleaning agents that strip away moisture and protective barriers of your skin, hair and mouth, which can cause dull, frizzy hair, possible follicular damage, potential hair loss, oral sores and dry skin. Governmental agencies consider sulfates to be safe ingredients; however, during the manufacturing process (known as *ethoxylation*), SLS/SLES becomes contaminated with 1,4 dioxane, a carcinogenic (cancer-causing) by-product. Health officials say that the small amount of this exposure does not affect health, nor has it been proven to cause cancer. Manufacturers do attempt to clean out the 1,4 dioxane by-product, but when it comes to your health, why take the risk? By choosing sulfate-free products, you may not enjoy the high-lather bubbles, but your hair, skin and mouth will enjoy a more natural, less abrasive, and long-term healthier appearance. I recommend choosing products with the USDA Organic Seal and an ingredients list you can pronounce. Ultimately, you have to research your products and make the best decisions for yourself and your family.

This chapter only discusses the tip of the iceberg here in regards to the hidden chemicals we use everyday. With so much exposure to many chemicals on a daily basis, and with the industry lacking regulation, it's up to the consumer to get informed and make the necessary changes. The first action step would be to take stock of your products and go to the Environmental Working Group's website (www.EWG.org) to search the toxicity of your items. This nonprofit provides a very user-friendly way to see how toxic or non-toxic your products are, as well as giving you the name of products and/or brands that are better options. As you run out of your toxic items, just replace them with non-toxic, healthier products. Even if you live in a rural area, it is very easy to order these items online now. You must learn to become a label reader and be your own health advocate.

Toxins in Your Cosmetics?

Toxic & Carcinogenic Compounds to Avoid

BENZOYL PEROXIDE
Found in: Acne products
Effects: Promotes skin tumors and premature skin aging

DEA-REGULATED INGREDIENTS (DIETHANOLAMINE, ETC.)
Found in: Foam booster such as shampoos, cosmetics, soaps and detergents
Effects: Skin/eye irritation and dermatitis

DIOXIN
Found in : Antibacterial ingredients
Effects: Cancer, reduces immunity, nervous system disorders, birth deformity, and miscarriages

FRAGRANCES
Found in: Found in everything from shampoo to deodorant
Effects: Cancer, allergies, asthma and neurotoxicity

FORMALDEHYDE & TOLUENE
Found in: Nail polish and ingredients in bath products
Effects: A known cancer-causing carcinogen

HEAVY METALS (LEAD, MERCURY I.E. THIMEROSOL)
Found in: Lipstick, men's hair coloring kits and cosmetics like mascara
Effects: Potent neurotoxicants that can damage overall human health

PHTHALATES
Found in: Classified as a pesticide. Not listed on labels and usually found in many products
Effects: Damage to liver/kidneys, birth defects, decreased sperm counts & early breast development in girls & boys

TRICLOSAN
Found in: Synthetic antibacterial ingredients labeled as a pesticide
Effects: Poses risks to human health and environment. Classified as a chlorophenol (chemicals suspected of causing cancer in humans)

Green America. "9 Toxins to Avoid in Personal Care Products." Green American, April/May 2011.
http://www.greenamerica.org/pubs/greenamerican/articles/MarAprMay2011/Nine-Toxins-to-avoid-in-personal-care-products.cfm?gclid=COWY-ar7_sACFVJo7Aod0joA-g
David Suzuki Foundation. "'Dirty Dozen' cosmetic chemicals to avoid." http://www.davidsuzuki.org/issues/health/science/toxics/dirty-dozen-cosmetic-chemicals/

I believe we need to seek wisdom in these matters of health and move forward with informed and health-conscious choices to prevent disharmony and disease in our bodies. I know God desires us to be healthy, but health doesn't just happen. As we gain knowledge of how we care for our bodies and what we subject them to on a daily basis, we can align ourselves closer to the natural laws of the body and become more congruent with God's design.

Cassandra Cutchens

I am one of six children. When all of us were younger, the joke was that I was the runt (true) and the sickly one (also true), so maybe I needed to be "put down" like they do in other litters. Sadly, I laughed with my siblings because it was so true.

As a child, I was diagnosed with mitral-valve prolapse, a heart defect. It was explained that I would always be under a cardiologist's care for this condition. I had to pre-medicate with antibiotics before any procedures and always before going to the dentist. My father had heart concerns, so I was prepared to always have heart issues just like him. At 12 years old, I was diagnosed with migraines. Over the next couple of years, I had a lot of tests to determine what was triggering them; however, I never got an answer. What I did get was a new prescription with each new specialist. I had two to three prescriptions and was still taking over-the-counter medications as well. Not only was I a hormonally distraught teenager at the time, but the medications made me feel constantly moody.

Over the next few years, I was diagnosed as a "chemical diabetic" and taken off all sugar for a while. Cutting out sugar did not change anything, so I was able to eat my sweets again (yippee!). Then I was diagnosed as having hyperthyroidism. I was always thin for my height, and according to the doctor this disease had to be the cause. The solution that they gave my mom was the use of radiation to destroy part of my thyroid, just enough to slow it down some. Immediately, my mom told them that she did not like that option and did not think she could agree to that. All of her children were thin, and it just did not sound reasonable to her. The doctors sent me off with another prescription to try to correct my thyroid, telling me it would just take longer to work.

By this time, I was accustomed to taking a new drug for whatever symptom arose. The migraines were getting worse and more frequent. I had started having nightmares that would wake me up, so I was not getting good sleep. I had spent some time in the hospital having tests to see if they could determine once and for all what was causing the migraines. Medically, there was still not an answer. I was told that the only thing to do was to take the meds and hope for the best.

By my early twenties, I was married with two children, and my health concerns were only getting worse. In between my first two children, I had a bad car accident and shattered my left forearm. Both bones were put back together with metal plates and screws. When my arm was "totally healed," I had a permanent weather predictor to show for it. At this point, I was taking all kinds of medications for all kinds of diagnoses. I was told that I was in danger of having high blood pressure, which would complicate my mitral valve prolapse, so I needed to start taking high blood pressure medication too. I was so down about my health, I couldn't even imagine how it could get any worse. I still had the migraines and was up to four prescriptions; when those didn't work, I started to get shots that would put me to sleep for days, so I was literally sleeping the migraine off! Often, I would forget to take something because

there were so many pills. My health made my life miserable—
and it only got worse.

I had started to have heavy menstrual cycles and some wicked
cramps (before this, my periods had been three to five days and
fairly regular). My cycle was very late, and my husband and I
had started to suspect that I was pregnant again. I took a test,
and it was positive. While we were not planning on getting
pregnant, we were still excited. I called for an appointment with
my doctor and scheduled it a couple of weeks out. Before the
appointment, I had started to cramp again severely. Then one
day, I began to bleed out. I was home alone with my toddlers,
so I had to wait for someone to come sit with them and then get
to the doctor. I found out I had a miscarriage, which no woman
ever wants to hear. I remember thinking to myself, *Great...now
I can't even do this right!* I went back to the doctor for a follow-
up a few weeks later, and I had continued sporadically bleeding,
which led to valid concerns that something was very wrong.
I endured many tests and an emotional roller coaster, while
trying to keep my marriage together, make my children happy,
and hang on to my job.

Ultimately, I was diagnosed with endometriosis. The
cause of endometriosis is unknown. One theory is that the
endometrial tissue is deposited in unusual locations by the
backing up of menstrual flow into the fallopian tubes and the
pelvic/abdominal cavity during menstruation. The result is
excessive bleeding and unbearable cramping. I was told that I
would never be able to carry a child full term again and that the
only solution was to have a hysterectomy. I had seen my mom
suffer with the same thing and knew this had to be hereditary.

She also had a hysterectomy, as had most of the women in my family, so I was not surprised by this forthcoming surgery.

What did surprise me is while we were trying to figure out the best time to schedule my hysterectomy, we found out I was pregnant again. At my next doctor's appointment, my husband and I were told that I could not carry the baby full term, so they advised us to have a medically necessary abortion and then go ahead with the hysterectomy as planned. They were also concerned with my mental stability if I tried to carry the baby and then lost it. Despite everything, our faith told us that God was in control of everything, and we needed to turn over our circumstances to Him. We let the doctors know that if anybody removed that baby from the womb, it would be the good Lord above, not a man. To my doctor's surprise, I did carry the baby full term and delivered her the old-fashioned way—no drugs or interventions, just laboring and pushing!

A few months after my daughter's birth, my symptoms returned, and I agreed to the hysterectomy at the age of 30. I was told I would gain 40 to 50 pounds and would need supplemental hormones, but all else would be "normal." I thought this was my answer, and I would start to feel better.

I did not.

All of my health concerns from before were still present, I did gain weight, *and* I developed new health concerns. I had begun to have seasonal allergies that turned into bronchitis that turned into pneumonia, which occurred two to three times a year. After several episodes like this, I began having severe chest pains, and thought I must be having my first heart attack. At the hospital, we found out it was pleurisy. I would have several cycles like this over the next few years, not knowing if it was my heart or my lungs each time. I now had no hope of ever feeling better and often worried about what my children would do when I was gone. I had given up.

One day my mom called me and said she had found a doctor that could help me with my migraines. She told me all about Dr. Hess and that she knew I would feel better if I would go. I had given up on that notion, so I delayed as long as I could. Finally, I went—but only after another car accident.

The first thing Dr. Hess told me was that having a headache every day was not normal. I argued that for me, it was normal. She taught me that my body was designed to heal itself, and if you remove the nerve interference, it could. She explained that the nerve interference could be the cause of many of my health concerns and that chiropractic care could help. She explained that God had made my body and God would heal my body; she was just going to remove the interference. At this point in my life, I felt like I tried everything else and nothing had worked, so what did I have to lose by giving chiropractic a chance?

I started to get adjustments, and soon my head did not hurt as often. As I continued, my migraines were fewer and fewer, and I was not taking as many pills. The Hesses continued to educate me on how God had designed my body and what it was able to do, if it was allowed to do it. We had a conversation about how the drugs could be causing harm to my body. I had never thought about it that way. When doctors write you a prescription, they always tell you how great the drug is for you. During this process, I realized that many of my health concerns were caused by some of the medications I was taking for other health concerns. I had been medicating my side effects for years! I began to wean off of the drugs as quickly as I could, and I stayed under care with Dr. Hess and allowed my body to heal the way it was designed to. Through this process, my hope was restored that I could be well again and have the quality of life that I was intended to have.

For several years now, I have been drug-free. I have lost my permanent "weather predictor," I do not have migraines every day, and all of my health concerns are nearly non-existent. I was even told by my cardiologist that I no longer have mitral valve prolapse, which is truly a miracle because that just does not happen. I had come to the point where I had to make a choice. I could continue medicating myself, probably undergo more tests and surgeries, and continue to be in a state of health misery, or I could say, *Enough is enough! I have been given medicine and pharmaceuticals 30-plus years of my life, and things are just getting worse! I've got to do things differently.* This is not to say that my health is perfect, but I am no longer the sick, over-medicated girl of my youth. I am a vibrant woman in her 40s who is healthier now than ever, and why? Because the Power that made the body heals my body!

3.

Tickled Pink
for Men in White

The typical conversation goes like this:

"Great specific adjustment today. I'll see you next week." As I am almost out of the room, my client replies, "Oh, Dr. Hess, I won't be in for about six weeks or so, because I'm having a female procedure done…" This is where I usually inquire which type of surgery, and the conversation generally moves in a predictable direction: why the client's doctor said she needed this female procedure and the justification for it.

When I first started in practice about 15 years ago, these conversations didn't really faze me. I knew that most of these women weren't aware that there were natural alternatives and other options, because either their M.D. never talked about or didn't know about them, or the women themselves never asked about or did their own research on the subject. But as the years have gone by, these discussions started to have a bigger effect on me, only because they kept happening and at an alarmingly increased rate. More and more women would tell me about procedures, further diagnostic testing, and necessary operations they had to have on their bodies "because their doctors said so," and quite frankly, the majority of them were absolutely convinced it was necessary—no questions asked!

As I continued to have these kinds of discussions with different women, I wondered if similar issues are in my future as well, and I asked myself what I could do differently so that I won't become this same story. This led me to my own research, and I started to find out staggering, even shocking, statistics. For example, the number one surgery performed on women is a cesarean section, with 33 percent of women in the United States now delivering their babies by cutting through the abdomen and uterus. That means one out of three women will be subjected to major abdominal surgery, a drawn-out recovery time, possible adhesions, a weakened uterine wall, and other side effects.

Yes, you might think of someone who needed a life-saving cesarean section surgery, and yes, some of these surgeries are necessary. However, according to the World Health Organization, cesarean section rates of five to ten percent are considered optimal and have the best outcomes for mom and baby.[1] Not to mention, there are many known benefits to having your baby vaginally, such as: a lower risk of respiratory problems such as asthma; the ability to receive protective bacteria as the baby passes through the birth canal to assist in the development of a balanced immune system; increased alertness if the delivery was drug-free; and easier skin-to-skin contact and attachment between mom and baby, just to name a few.

1. "Why Is the National U.S. Cesarean Section Rate So High?" Childbirth Connection. http://www.childbirthconnection.org/article.asp?ck=10456

To my dismay, the second most common surgery performed on women is a hysterectomy, removal of the uterus and/or other related female reproductive organs. This procedure has long-term, broad, negative ramifications to a woman's body, which many doctors may dismiss or routinely fail to mention. Research shows that "99.7 percent of women...were given little or no prior information about the acknowledged adverse effects of hysterectomy—information that is a legal requisite of consent."[2] The laundry list of negative effects after a hysterectomy is horrific, with 79 percent of women experiencing personality change and irritability, 77 percent encountering loss of energy and profound fatigue, 75 percent feeling diminished or absent sexual desire, 66 percent suffering bone and joint pain, 60 percent enduring insomnia, and 53 percent facing suicidal thoughts... just to name a few of the dozens of reported side effects![3] The sad truth is that a nonprofit women's health group named HERS (Hysterectomy Educational Resources and Services) stated that "98 percent of women [that] HERS has referred to board-certified gynecologists after being told they needed hysterectomies, discovered that, in fact, they did not need hysterectomies." Moreover, "Gynecologists, hospitals and drug companies make more than $17 billion dollars a year from the business of hysterectomy and castration."[4] That's right—castration, when the ovaries are removed during a hysterectomy, unfortunately occurring in 73 percent of all hysterectomies. In

2. Newman, Amie. "Overused and Underinformed: The Secrets of the Hysterectomy in the U.S." RH Reality Check. http://rhrealitycheck.org/article/2010/05/19/overused-underinformed-secrets-hysterectomy/

3. "Adverse Effects Data." HERS Foundation. http://hersfoundation.org/effects.html

4. "Facts About Hysterectomy." HERS Foundation. http://hersfoundation.org/facts.html

the United States, one out of three women can be expected to have a hysterectomy by age 60.[5]

I clearly remember one dinner with family and friends about a year ago. We were eating homemade fajitas, Spanish rice and guacamole, and we all were having typical conversations, telling my mother how great her cooking was, listening to my father talk about his golf game and discussing the kids and their activities. One of the women suddenly confided that she was scheduled for her hysterectomy later that week—just in time so that it wouldn't interfere with the kids' spring break. Having known this person my entire life and also knowing that I probably wasn't going to change her mind, I recognized that this was my only chance to say anything before her surgery. So, in keeping with my straightforward personality, I said, "Look, you probably don't want to hear my opinion on this, but I'm going to give it anyway. A hysterectomy is a major surgery with known significant side effects. Have you considered a second opinion on this? Have you researched natural alternatives to get your hormones and reproductive system back to homeostasis and a balanced state? Your symptoms are a reflection of an underlying problem, and I really think you should explore some other options before consenting to this surgery."

Women are more diagnosed, more drugged, and more cut on than men.

I then received the response I expected. "Amanda, it [the uterus] has served its purpose. You just don't understand. I'm

---

5. "Hysterectomy Fact Sheet." Office on Women's Health, U.S. Department of Health and Human Services. http://www.womenshealth.gov/publications/our-publications/fact-sheet/hysterectomy.html.

bleeding continuously and it's not stopping. My hemoglobin levels are low, and I just don't have time for all this natural stuff you always talk about." So I got up from the dinner table and said, "Well, you're right. If you don't want to investigate other options, then you should definitely have your hysterectomy."

Why is it that so many of us fall prey to covering up or masking our health problems and sicknesses with pharmaceutical drugs and surgery? As God's creations, we can't forget that every time we look past the cause of the problem and just cover up the symptoms, we are cheating ourselves of having the life and health that God desires for us. A recent national survey from Loyola University's Stritch School of Medicine found that women were three times more likely to see a doctor on a regular basis than men.[6] It would only make sense, then, that women are more diagnosed, more drugged and more cut on than men. It seems that almost every woman who enters my office is either on an antidepressant or anti-anxiety medication. I believe that our culture has convinced us that we need to be "happy" with the perfect marriage, the perfect job, the perfect house and the perfect family. We see images, advertisements, TV series and movies portraying "the way things should be." As a culture in pursuit of this image-oriented happiness, should we be proud of the fact that research now shows that one in four women are on antidepressants and mental health drugs?[7] Are 25 percent of us so deficient in our mental capabilities that we need a pill every day to function?

6. Kevin Polsley, MD. "Man up – see a doctor." Loyola University Health System. http://www.loyolahealthyliving.org/2012/09/07/man-up-see-a-doctor/

7. Bindley, Katherine. "Women and Perscription Drugs: One in Four Takes Mental Health Meds." *Huffington Post*. http://www.huffingtonpost.com/2011/11/16/women-and-prescription-drug-use_n_1098023.html

Six months ago, a lady who had been seeing me for chiropractic care was raving about how her headaches had diminished, her chronic neck and back pain (from lifting heavy animals as a veterinary technician) had improved, and she was sleeping more soundly. I asked her if she was able to reduce any of her medications, and she said that it had been over a month since she had to take Imitrex for a migraine, and her Excedrin intake went from every day, multiple times per day, to just maybe one or two times per week. I congratulated her and then asked if she was taking anything else.

She then said she was on an antidepressant. I was surprised and told her that she always seemed so upbeat to me. I asked her how long she had been taking the antidepressant. She said that she began it during some marital troubles and after the death of her mother, which was five years ago. I

During the course of my Prozac intake, I wasn't the beautiful woman on the television or magazine advertisements thrilled with my Prozac.

acknowledged that it must have been a tough time for her, dealing with a lot of stress. When I asked her how everything was now, she responded that everything was great, so I inquired if she thought she still needed the antidepressant, or if she had talked to her doctor about it. Five years was a long time; was she going to have to take it for the rest of her life? Instantly, this woman had a revelation. She said, "You know what? You're absolutely right. I don't want to be taking this for the rest of my life. I need to call my doctor next week and talk about getting me off this stuff."

Another couple of months went by, and during one of her appointments with me, she said to me, "I want to thank you for encouraging me about that antidepressant. I have been weaning myself off of it, but let me tell you. I had no idea that the withdrawal symptoms would be so bad. I've been having these brain zaps, which are a known withdrawal symptom when someone comes off of antidepressants. If I had known it was going to be this bad, I would have never taken the stuff in the first place."

I also remember being a young 20-year-old in college, feeling stressed out, dealing with some addictions and having many uncertainties about my future. During a routine visit to the man in the white coat, he prescribed me Prozac. I blindly trusted this diagnosis and was actually excited that this pill was going to help me. Not researching the host of side effects of Prozac (including sexual dysfunction, dry mouth, nausea, headache, diarrhea, nervousness, restlessness, agitation, increased sweating, weight changes, insomnia and drowsiness), I began taking my dosage diligently. During the course of my Prozac intake, I wasn't the beautiful woman on the television or magazine advertisements thrilled with my Prozac. I began to have erratic behavior; I suffered some major hallucinations; and it was also the only time in my life that I dealt with suicidal thoughts. Upon getting off the Prozac, I dealt with excessive sweating over the next year, especially while sleeping. I would wake up with my clothes and my sheets wet from my sweat. I thank God that He brought my husband into my life at that critical time, as he was instrumental in supporting me and helping me through that year of withdrawal. Looking back now, I am thankful for these trials in my life, as I believe they have helped shape me into the person I am today. I should have informed myself prior to consenting, but we all learn from our mistakes.

As a follower of Jesus Christ, what also troubles me is the amount of women, men and children in churches who are on antidepressants or mental health drugs. When we claim that there is "power in the blood of Jesus" and the Holy Spirit is our Comforter and Deliverer, why then is such a large percentage of the body of Christ using mental health drugs? It's a tough subject to discuss, but just as the church at large is tackling the over 50 percent divorce rate among Christians, they should also question and discuss the overutilization of mental health drugs—and pharmaceuticals in general—among believers. Let's not forget, the word *pharmakia* literally means "drugs" and appears five times in the New Testament: Galatians 5:20, and Revelation 9:21,18:23, 21:8 and 22:15. *Pharmakia* is also translated into our English Bible as either "witchcraft" or "sorceries". We derive our English word "pharmacy" from the same word.[8]

Where do we go from here? What can I, or any of us, possibly say after looking at the grim facts—other than to see the gift of grace that God gave through his Son, Jesus Christ, and to acknowledge that our joy comes from being in His presence. In His presence is strength, joy, and knowledge. Knowledge is the first of many steps in removing as many pharmaceuticals as possible from the church and our lives. I believe women can be victorious in their quest for health, and I believe there is a

8. "On the Greek word "pharmakia." True Discernment. http://truediscernment.com/2007/07/09/on-the-greek-word-pharmakia/

Downsides of Hysterectomy

99.7% of women...were given little or no prior information about the acknowledged adverse effects of hysterectomy—information that is a legal requisite of consent.

98% of women [that] HERS (Hysterectomy Educational Resources and Services) has referred to board-certified gynecologists after being told they needed hysterectomies, discovered that, in fact, they did not need hysterectomies.

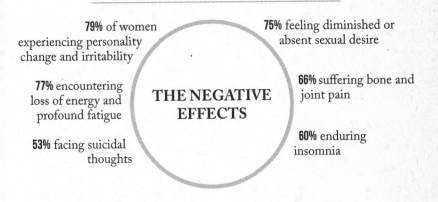

79% of women experiencing personality change and irritability

77% encountering loss of energy and profound fatigue

53% facing suicidal thoughts

THE NEGATIVE EFFECTS

75% feeling diminished or absent sexual desire

66% suffering bone and joint pain

60% enduring insomnia

One out of three women can be expected to have a hysterectomy by age 60 in the United States.

"Adverse Effects Data." HERS Foundation. http://hersfoundation.org/effects.html

Newman, Amie. "Overused and Underinformed: The Secrets of the Hysterectomy in the U.S." RH Reality Check. http://rhrealitycheck.org/article/2010/05/19/over-used-underinformed-secrets-hysterectomy/

"Hysterectomy Fact Sheet." Office on Women's Health, U.S. Department of Health and Human Services. http://www.womenshealth.gov/publications/our-publications/fact-sheet/hysterectomy.html.

better way, a right way, for women to claim their God-given birthright of true health from the inside out. Women must rise up, ask questions, become informed and take responsibility for their health.

Mimi Howe

How do you write down forty years of your life in just a few pages? I guess I will start with the highlights. When I was eleven years old, I began passing blood. Within six weeks the doctors had diagnosed me with ulcerative colitis. This would explain the pain I had lived with for as long as I could remember. I remember telling my mom that my stomach hurt. Like most moms, she thought I just had a tummy ache. When the doctors gave me the diagnosis, they immediately went into their version of "cure" mode; if we remove the colon, then the problem is gone. Thank God my mother was a thinking woman and decided that if removing my colon ever needed to happen, it should be my decision and not hers. As you're reading this, please understand that this was long before the Internet or search engines. We had limited information about the medical route of treatment or the natural/holistic route.

I lived with monstrous pain from not only the colitis, but also from the steroids and the kidney stones that my condition, the prescribed medications, and my diet created. The gastroenterologist gave me a low-residue diet to follow. This diet consisted of canned foods, no fiber, white processed breads, white potatoes and straight sugar. Dairy was removed as well.

I was in and out of hospitals for the next thirty years, either ill or being tested, drugged or biopsied. I was in a constant state of fatigue. The doctors told me that I wouldn't live past the age of fifty, that my bones would be so curled up from the steroids that I would be bent over at an almost ninety degree angle, and I would die childless. After years of medical care, my situation was not improving and my prognosis appeared hopeless.

When I met and married my husband at the age of 32, he tried to tell me there was a better way to health. He had grown up in a home where natural remedies and chiropractic care were the first lines of defense against any illness. I had been in the medical community since I was a child. I considered myself a know-it-all and wasn't going to budge. It took a horrible childbirth experience to convince me to go in a different direction.

My water broke the evening of May 7, 1992. I called my doctor and immediately headed to the hospital. When I arrived, I was placed in a bed and attached to monitors. Although I wasn't in much pain, the nurse insisted that the pain would get much worse, and I needed a shot to thwart the pain. Although I was telling myself not to do it, I complied and allowed them to give it to me. Then my troubles began. My labor stopped, and since my water was already broken, they immediately started the induction of labor with Pitocin. During the hardest point of my labor, my doctor left me for another baby in distress and didn't return until my baby was in distress. I was forced into an emergency Cesarean section. I woke up sore from pushing, along with torn musculature, a terrible incision from the Cesarean, and blindness. I did not opt for an epidural, so in the process of putting me to sleep for the emergency Cesarean section surgery, the anesthesiologist taped my eyes shut, forgetting to close them before they were taped. When they removed the tape, they also removed the top layer of my eyes. I know this sounds unbelievable, but the story does not end here. Upon waking up two days later from the overdose of anesthesia, I found out that my baby had not been fed anything. What in the world was going on?

Now blind and still in a stupor from the anesthesia, I tried to breastfeed my daughter. The ophthalmologist believed that my sight would return because it was a superficial wound. After a horrible labor, incisions through my abdomen and uterus from the Cesarean section, anesthesia overdose, waking up blind, and learning that my baby had not been fed anything, that's when I began to question the medical community.

Over the next few months I had a hard time lifting my baby because of the muscle strains in my arms, hands and thumbs from the writhing in labor. My back went out on me regularly, with me flat on the floor not moving for hours trying to relieve the pain. I depended on family to watch my child because I couldn't do it myself. One day, my sister and my husband took me to a chiropractor. I knew all the horror stories and had been told that chiropractors were quacks.

Fearful with no belief in chiropractic, but willing to try anything at this point, I was amazed at how I felt after my first adjustment. My hips had been out of alignment for so long that I honestly believed one leg was shorter than the other. I even walked that way. I continued on my chiropractic journey. I had already given the medical community 30-plus years of my life, so it only made sense to give chiropractic time to help me function better. The most amazing part was that my general health started improving as well. No one ever explained to me how chiropractic worked and it didn't really matter. I just assumed it was to make my back pain go away, which it did, but I was pleased that I had fewer and fewer flare-ups of my colitis over the next year.

Years later, after witnessing my parents' diagnosis of Alzheimer's disease and helping to keep my father alive on a feeding tube for *nine years* in hospice care, I became voracious with the study of the human body. Yes, you read that right. My father was in hospice care for nine years. I do believe that's a record! I learned that chiropractic focuses on the nervous system, which controls and enhances every function of the body. I learned that fresh fruits and vegetables did no harm to an ulcerated colon. I learned that our body becomes depleted in vitamins, minerals, enzymes, and amino acids by what we do to it, emotionally and physically. I learned that our bodies needed and could be replenished naturally.

My children grew up, like my husband, with natural remedies and chiropractic care as their first lines of defense. My health is much better now than in my youth, and you will always find me and my family "encouraging" or "arguing" with others to seek the natural route to health. People perish for a lack of knowledge, and I am thankful for the trials as well as the triumphs with my health.

Mimi Howe
Columbus, GA
Wife, Mother, Grandmother

4.

Body Built for a Baby

Dr. Amanda Hess and Charity Haulk

It never ceases to amaze me how God designed us, built us and prepared us for greatness. Even looking at Genesis chapter 2, the Creation story tells us that God made man and woman in His own image. It describes how He blessed them, telling them to be fruitful and multiply, to fill the Earth, govern it and reign over all the animals. When God created Adam, He placed him in the garden to tend and watch over it. But God said, "It is not good for man to be alone," so He made him a helper just right for him. After causing Adam to fall into a deep sleep, God took out one of his ribs, and from the rib created woman. When God brought her to Adam, he was so excited, exclaiming, "At last, this one is from my bone, and flesh of my flesh! She will be called *woman*, because she was taken from man."

The Creation story reminds us that even though we cannot always see how our bodies are created on the inside, we can have faith that from the beginning of the world, God has designed our bodies with all the parts necessary to live, thrive and reproduce. Men and women create children together, but only women have the special ability to house and birth life. Woman is unique in her design; internally and externally, she is shaped and formed differently from man. Women also have three very important physiological functions, which are totally absent in men: *menstruation, pregnancy* and *lactation*. I find it fascinating to see how each part of our bodies serves a specific and unique purpose, and I believe understanding their purpose will not only give clarity to how and why they work the way they do, but also inspire us to nurture and take care of these special "womanly" aspects God has graced us with.

I believe that part of the purpose of every woman's life is to rear children and pave the way for the next generation. While not every woman bears children, each can have their own part in bringing out the best traits, characteristics and qualities in any child. Moreover, every woman can advocate the belief that God gave us and our bodies everything we need to make the process of birthing a baby natural, effective, and fearless.

> Every woman can advocate the belief that God gave us and our bodies everything we need to make the process of birthing a baby natural, effective, and fearless.

In one common medical situation, a doctor informs a woman her pelvis is "too small or inadequate," or the baby is thought to be "too big" to birth, so she is advised to have a cesarean section. Whenever I hear these statements, I have to control myself to not explode with emotion. How could a woman's own body, fueled by its innate intelligence, possibly build and create a baby inside of her that is too big to birth through her pelvic birth canal? The medical term for this diagnosis is cephalopelvic disproportion, or CPD. However, research indicates that pelvimetry, which is the commonly used procedure to measure the pelvis, is not a useful diagnostic tool for CPD, and in all cases, trial of labor should be allowed.[1]

I clearly remember the distress of a young woman who was pregnant for the first time. She had been told that her baby was measuring over 10 pounds, and there was no way her petite pelvis could birth this baby naturally. She felt defeated and questioned why God would have created her body not to be able to handle the birth of her baby. After the scheduled cesarean section, she was delighted to have a healthy baby, but upset that she allowed herself to not believe in God's perfect design of her body when her baby was born at only 8 pounds, 2 ounces. For her next birth, she chose to believe in herself and had a VBAC (vaginal birth after cesarean) of her 8 pound, 6 ounce baby.

Colossians 2:19 says, "Christ gives the body its strength, and He uses its joints and muscles to hold it together, as it grows by the power of God." Many women falsely believe that their pelvis capacity is limited, and therefore, that they will have difficulty in giving birth. The good news is that God created specific ligaments, muscles, organs and hormones that all assist each other in the normal functioning of a woman. During pregnancy, these muscles and ligaments provide support to the bladder, bowels and uterus. In childbirth, they help guide the baby's head down through the birth canal. The hormone relaxin softens many of these ligaments, allowing the uterus and pelvis to expand as the baby grows. It also relaxes the arteries to help with the higher blood volume and to loosen

1. Blackadar, C.S. and A. Viera: "A Retrospective Review of Performance and Uitlity of Routine Clinical Pelvimetry." *AAFP* 2003, 36(7), 505.

up the musculoskeletal system, allowing increased curvature in the back in preparation for carrying and delivering a baby. [2]

Many women like myself will (on several occasions and without any warning) experience these sharp groin pains, which are ligament pains, as the baby grows, expands and moves. For whatever reason (probably instinctively), I would always fall to the ground and begin kneeling and tilting my pelvis, which would provide immediate relief. Pregnant woman should seek chiropractic care to utilize the benefits of keeping the pelvis and lower spine in proper balance and free of nerve interference for the best birth possible. In our chiropractic practice, we see dozens of pregnant women every week to help them alleviate all types of pain and ailments that can surface during pregnancy. It's such a joy to hear story after story of natural births with shorter than normal labor times, less invasive procedures and the emphasis placed on the woman's natural ability to do what it is built and designed by God to do.

> Many of the healthcare system's standard procedures weren't always the best practice—and definitely not the most natural.

As I became more aware of natural birthing methods with both of my pregnancies, I started to learn that many of the healthcare system's standard procedures weren't always the best practice—and definitely not the most natural. For example, when a woman labors on her back with her feet in stirrups, she is going in opposition to God's perfect design. Lying on your back places all the weight on the sacrum (tailbone area),

2. Dixon, Amy. "Pregnancy & Ligaments Stretching." Livestrong.com. http://www.livestrong.com/article/304142-pregnancy-ligaments-stretching/#ixzz2PjhDP1KT

narrowing the pelvic outlet. It compresses major blood vessels, lowering the oxygen supply to the baby and leading to fetal distress. It also will promote weaker, less frequent, and more irregular contractions, and instead of the baby naturally descending out of the birth canal from a mother's squatting position, now the baby has to ascend out of the birth canal, against gravity, in the lying down position.

Another statistic I encountered was the all-too-routine use of epidurals, with 75 percent of women in the United States reporting having an epidural during labor. In an epidural, a local anesthetic—a derivative of cocaine—is injected into the epidural space (the space around the tough coverings that protect the spinal cord). Epidurals block nerve signals from both the sensory and motor nerves, which provides effective pain relief, but also immobilizes the lower part of the woman's body. There are different types of epidurals, and each needs to be researched before any woman blindly subjects her body to one. There are many red flags here, but the big ones are:

1. Epidurals reduce oxytocin production, which slows down and lengthens birth
2. Epidurals triple the rate of severe perineal tearing
3. Epidurals increase the risk of C-section by two and a half times
4. Epidurals triple the occurrence of induction of birth with Pitocin
5. Epidurals increase the risk of urinary, anal and sexual disorders in mothers after birth

6. Epidurals may interfere with mother-baby bonding and breastfeeding
7. Epidurals interfere with the normal hormonal production during the labor and delivery process[3]

There are many effective and natural techniques that can assist a woman in a natural birth. For example, the perineum is the area of skin between the rectum and the vagina. During labor, these muscles stretch around the baby's head as he or she comes out of the vaginal canal. A mother can start doing perineal massages as early as six weeks before labor. These daily massages will stretch and prepare the skin of the perineum for birth. The extra advantage of performing perineal massage may allow the mother to give birth without an episiotomy—a surgical incision in the posterior vaginal wall, from the vulva to the anus.

> Anytime we add medications or epidurals to the birthing process, we increase the chance of complications and adverse reactions.

My friend Cristina had an emergency cesarean section for her first baby after a routine checkup at 38 weeks, during which the OBGYN discovered her baby was in a breech position. Her recovery from the cesarean was not pleasant, and she wanted a VBAC for her second child. It took quite a bit of searching for the right provider who would support her in this decision. A few days before her due date of her second child, I remember getting a voicemail from Cristina, and it was very apparent that she was having some fear and anxiety with her

3. Kresser, Chris. "Natural childbirth V: epidural side effects and risks." http://chriskresser.com/natural-childbirth-v-epidural-side-effects-and-risks

upcoming due date. When I called her back, she didn't answer, so I just left her a message and prayed for her.

As it turned out, Cristina was successful in having a VBAC; however, it included an unwanted episiotomy following her medicated birth of induction drugs and epidural anesthesia. While she was happier with this outcome, after about eight weeks, things just weren't right. She called me asking for my opinion, because she was having excruciating pain whenever she went to the bathroom. She said even the slightest touch of toilet paper produced a pain that she said was beyond description. She was further concerned because there was no way she could resume sexual relations with her husband. She wasn't sure if this was normal and wanted my thoughts on the matter; I told her to call her OBGYN the next day and get an appointment immediately, because the type of pain she was describing was definitely not normal. As it turned out, Cristina had a flap of skin (from her inside) hanging on the outside of her, sewn incorrectly after her episiotomy, which was causing her severe pain. Her OBGYN removed it, and she is thankful to be doing much better now.

Anytime we add medications or epidurals to the birthing process, we increase the chance of complications and adverse reactions, as was also the case with my friend Charity's first birth. Toward the end of her son's birth, his shoulders got stuck (also known as shoulder dystocia). Because she was paralyzed from the epidural and lying flat on her back unable to move, she could not get into a position that would help free his shoulders. When Ethan went into fetal distress, she was given an episiotomy to free his shoulders while the vacuum extractor was attached to his skull, forcefully pulling him out of the birth canal. On the other hand, when she gave birth naturally (un-medicated) with her daughter, Lauren, her midwife administered perineal massage during the entire birth. When Lauren was born, she weighed 8 pounds, 12 ounces—a pound more than Ethan. Charity barely tore and did not need any stitches. All Charity had to do was make sure she did not sit cross-legged, instead keeping her legs straight to help the tear heal. When she gave birth naturally to her son Hayden, *he* weighed 9 pounds, 12 ounces! Again, she barely tore and did not need stitches.

During Charity's first birth with Ethan, she thought a drug-induced, pain-free delivery was the best option for her and her baby; however, by going against God's natural, physiological mechanisms of the body, Ethan's birth was the most traumatic, not only for Charity but also for her baby. For her next two deliveries, she utilized chiropractic care regularly, was purposeful about what she ate and put into her body, and decided to trust in God's design and allow her body to function naturally without any pharmaceuticals. She felt every contraction, every ounce of pain, and successfully birthed her other two children naturally and more easily than her first medicated birth.

Most of you have heard of the "love hormone" oxytocin. Oxytocin is the natural hormone released by the mother during childbirth. This love hormone is released by both men and women during orgasm, as well as with mother and baby as they bond during breastfeeding. The synthetic form of oxytocin is Pitocin. It is administered intravenously, and the dosage can be monitored and increased, decreased or stopped at anytime. Pitocin is used to induce labor, strengthen labor contractions during childbirth, control bleeding after childbirth or to induce an abortion. Pitocin-induced contractions will be longer, more forceful and much closer together than a woman's natural contractions. This can cause significant stress to the baby, because there's not enough time to recover from the reduced blood flow from the placenta, which compresses with each contraction. The net effect of this is to deprive the baby of necessary supplies of blood and oxygen, which can in turn lead to abnormal fetal heart rate patterns and fetal distress.[4]

Pitocin also does not give the mother a natural break between contractions. Furthermore, the contractions are so strong that the mother is unable to cope with the unnatural and severe pain, so she is given an epidural so that she won't be able to feel any of it, but this in turn may lead to the cascade of side effects from the epidural. Thus, the interventions continue. Common side effects of Pitocin include fetal heart abnormalities (slow heart beat, PVCs and arrhythmias), low APGAR scores, neonatal jaundice, neonatal retinal hemorrhage, permanent central nervous system or brain damage, and fetal death. A Swedish study showed a nearly 3 times greater risk of asphyxia (oxygen deprivation) for babies born after augmentation with Pitocin.[5] And a study in Nepal showed that induced babies were 5 times more likely to have signs of brain damage at birth.[6] In fact,

4. Stubbs, TM. "Oxytocin for labor induction." *Clinical Obstetrics and Gynecology* September 2000, 43(3), 489-94.

5. Ladfors L, Milsom I, Niklasson A, Odeback A, Thiringer K and E Thornberg. "Influence of maternal, obstetric and fetal risk factors on the prevalence of birth asphyxia at term in a Swedish urban population." *Acta Obstetricia et Gynecologica Scandinavica* October 2002, 81(10), 909-17.

6. Ellis, Matthew. "Risk factors for neonatal encephalopathy in Kathmandu, Nepal, a developing country: unmatched case-control study." *British Medical Journal* May 6, 2000, 320(7244), 1229-1236.

birth activist Doris Haire describes the effects of synthetic oxytocin on the baby as follows:

> *"The situation is analogous to holding an infant under the surface of the water, allowing the infant to come to the surface to gasp for air, but not to breathe."[7]*

Pitocin can also cause complications for women both during and after childbirth. Evidence suggests that women who receive Pitocin have increased risk of postpartum hemorrhage, which is likely due to the prolonged exposure to non-pulsed oxytocin. This makes the oxytocin receptors in the uterus insensitive to oxytocin ("oxytocin resistance") and the woman's own postpartum oxytocin release ineffective in preventing hemorrhage after birth. Some studies also indicate that Pitocin may have effects on the natural hormonal cascade. Hormonal disruption may also explain the reduced rate of breastfeeding following labor that was induced with Pitocin. Pitocin can be a useful and even life-saving procedure, and should absolutely be used when necessary. However, the evidence suggests that it is not without side effects and risks, and it should not be used in routine or otherwise uncomplicated birth.

One of my favorite verses is James 1:17, which says, "Every good and perfect gift is from above, coming down from the Father of heavenly lights, who does not change like shifting shadows." When Jeremy and I give our children gifts for Christmas or their birthdays, we don't give them broken toys—we give them toys that work! Sometimes, the gifts we give

---

7. Haire, Doris. "Improving the Outcom of Pregnancy through Science." American Foundation for Maternal and Child Health. http://www.aimsusa.org/ImprovingThroughScience.htm

Epidurals

Major Side Effects & Risks

Reduce oxytocin production, which can slow down and lengthen labor.

Triple the rate of severe perineal tearing.

Increase the risk of C-section by two and a half times.

Triple the occurrence of induction of birth with Pitocin.

Increase the risk of urinary, anal and sexual disorders in mothers after birth.

May interfere with mother-baby bonding and breastfeeding.

Epidurals interfere with the normal hormonal production during the labor and delivery process.

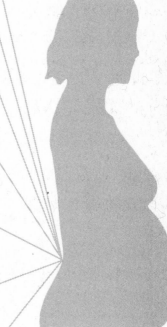

Kresser, Chris. "Natural childbirth V: epidural side effects and risks." http://chriskresser.com/natural-childbirth-v-epidural-side-effects-and-risks

them have to be put together so they can play with them. If they need batteries, we put them in so they will run and work properly. We want them to enjoy their toys and get the most out of them. God did the same thing for us at the beginning of Creation. His creation of the human body is perfectly designed; He didn't give us broken bodies that don't work properly, nor did He give us bodies not equipped with all the necessary parts. He has always been the same since the beginning of the world, and His design of our bodies has never changed. Women should cherish and embrace God's perfect design and realize that all the many parts of a woman's body serve a purpose each and every day of her life. A woman's body is designed with perfection for pregnancy and childbirth. Women need to realize that our bodies naturally function best if we'd honor "a body built for a baby."

Emily Ward

Unlike many couples first starting out, my husband and I knew in the beginning of marriage that we did not want to wait to have children. So, after getting married December 8th, 2012, we were overjoyed to find out on February 28th, 2013, that we were three weeks pregnant! We had done what we thought was a lot of research on pregnancy, labor, and child rearing, but in fact, it was not enough at all. However, we did know that we wanted an all-natural labor process. We looked around for the most natural ways of going about a hospital birth in the town we lived in, and one of the clinics offered medical midwifery instead of OB services. After looking at Internet reviews, we decided to set up an appointment. We went in for our first appointment and everyone was very nice. The nurse-midwife we met was agreeable with everything we wanted, so going home that day, we felt genuinely happy about our experience.

About that time, we were told about a weekly natural childbirth class that was being held at the Hesses' practice 85 miles away, and we made the journey because we thought it was that important. We loved all the information that Charity, the doula/educator, shared, and we made many decisions on issues that we previously hadn't even considered. Charity planned a fieldtrip to a meet-and-greet at Intown Midwifery in metro Atlanta, Georgia. The main speaker of the night would be Dr. Brad Bootstaylor, MD, FACOG, talking about his commitment to mothers having natural births, sharing how he was in support of homebirth, and discussing how he was now accepting homebirth transfers. We were encouraged to discover that there were MDs that fully support homebirth.

After numerous appointments at the clinic, we went in for a routine pregnancy check-up. Our primary midwife came into the room, with the typical introduction of, "How are you feeling? Do you have any questions?" After looking at my ultrasound and bringing up hospital protocol, she mentioned that induction procedures would occur after 41 weeks and 6 days. Puzzled, my husband and I looked at her, looked at each other and replied, "We don't plan on being induced." She responded, "Well, we'll just cross that bridge when we get to it."

It seemed that at every appointment, staff members at the clinic wanted to bring up some form of "hospital protocol" that they hadn't felt the need to share in all of the previous months of appointments. Now fully aware of all this, we had a decision to make: Would we want to have a planned homebirth and use the clinic for emergency/transfer care? Or, should we just stick to what we were doing and hope that nothing bad happened?

We had a clinic appointment on November 15th, which would have put me at 41 weeks and 4 days. We went to the Women's Center at the hospital affiliated with the clinic and headed straight in for an NST (fetal non-stress test) and ultrasound, which both came up normal as we had expected. When the nurse-midwife walked into the exam room, she seemed almost in a panic, mainly because our regular midwife was at a conference, and she didn't know much about our case.

She informed us that she was scheduling our induction for Sunday, November 17th, which would put me exactly at 41 weeks and 6 days. We explained that we had no expectations of inducing at all, and asked if there was any way for her to force us to do anything, to which she replied that she did not. She told us she would expect us to come in for a full induction on Sunday at 5 PM, but if we decided not to come, to come into the clinic Monday morning, as our regular midwife would be back from her trip.

On Monday morning, after (obviously) not showing up to our induction, we were met at the door of the clinic with angry faces, judgmental body language and arrogant tones. We were called back for an ultrasound, where the nurse-midwife told us that she didn't see enough fluid and my placenta was starting to die. We then were taken back to the NST, and while she pushed on my abdomen, she told us that my son's heartbeat was weak and losing beats by the second. She proceeded to try to push us into inducing that day, because it was her last day of the week "on call." After 45 minutes of her and my husband arguing back and forth about induction, she stood up and said, "Well maybe we should have the *mother* make this decision. Emily, what do you want for your baby?"

"I already told you, I'm not going to be induced," I replied, knowing that there was no reason to induce other than hospital protocol and firm in my belief that God was in control. She left the room and returned after another 45 minutes, now bringing with her a piece of paper stating that we were releasing the clinic from responsibility if anything were to happen to the baby. We gladly signed it and walked out.

Later on that day, my husband was talking to my father about getting a second opinion and making an appointment with Dr. Bootstaylor in Atlanta. Since this was Monday, November 18th, and I was 42 weeks on the button, we called the office and were able to set an appointment for the next day. The environment at his clinic was very comforting and welcoming to my family, who had accompanied us. They were accepting of our wishes for a natural birth and explained everything carefully, and then they did an NST and ultrasound. The ultrasound found a good amount of fluid. After 20 minutes on the NST, the nurse let me know that as long as the baby made at least 7 movements in an hour, he was doing great. So when we went in to discuss the NST and ultrasound with the doctor, he told us that our baby had moved well over 7 times in the 20 minute period, which was obviously good.

The next day, we had one more appointment at our original clinic. But when we arrived, we once again walked into whispers and angry looks. When we headed back to NST and the nurse came in, she started asking us why we weren't getting induced and then proceeded to tell us about a mother who was getting an NST, just like me, and she didn't want to get induced, just like me, and her blood pressure dropped to the point where the doctor had to rush in, pull his car around and take her to the hospital for an emergency C-section.

After the nurse left the room, my husband looked over at me and said, "Babe, I was looking at the numbers the entire time, and the measurement never went anywhere near what she was saying; it stayed in the acceptable range and the only time it dropped was when she was moving the device around." After that, we went to the ultrasound room, where, before the exam had even begun, the nurse started speculating on what they had said in Atlanta about my ultrasound there.

"I don't know what they saw on their machines yesterday, but I don't see the amount of fluid they found," she muttered. A different midwife then walked into the exam room and said, "I'm not going to beat around the bush, so we are just going to go ahead and cut to the chase. Your baby's heart rate dropped into the 60s for 8 minutes, so that's already a pretty bad sign. Basically what will happen is the fluid in your uterus is going to keep going down and your baby's blood pressure is going to drop and drop and drop until your baby dies. I don't know what their findings were yesterday at your appointment, but they're just wrong." She then stood up and instructed us, "Right now, I need you to just go over to the hospital for a full NST."

My husband responded, "After everything this morning and how long my wife has already been here today, she hasn't eaten at all and I believe she will start to get sick in a minute if she doesn't."

"Well, you obviously don't trust us here, and trust is a big thing, so you should just probably switch your care over to Dr. Bootstaylor's office. I'll call them after you get your NST," she said. To this I replied, "I've been here for many hours, and I need to get some food, because I am getting sick to my stomach. You can't just call over there now, because we are not going for the NST right now."

"I need to go to lunch so I can't call them right now, but I do need you to head over to the hospital for that monitoring, and if you have to eat, just run through a drive-through real quick and come back," she said.

"Well, my wife is 42 weeks pregnant, and I think it's kind of a big deal that she hasn't eaten yet, so we're going to do that before we do anything," said my husband as we walked out of the door. She looked at us puzzled because we were leaving and said, "Just get to the hospital before 4:30!"

That day was Mom's birthday, so we were meeting my family for lunch downtown. About 5 minutes into our meal, the clinic staff started blowing up our phones, and since we were with all the people that were our emergency contacts, their phones were being called too.

After about an hour of being harassed, we finally answered, only to hear the same fear tactics we were hearing before we left. We were so annoyed that we called Dr. Bootstaylor and asked him if we could switch care to them, since we needed to get away from the clinic because they would not accept our birth plan. He said he had been trying to get in touch with them the whole day.

I walked over to my husband as he put his phone on speaker, just in time for us to hear the midwife say that she had been trying to call Dr. Bootstaylor for a couple hours and he wouldn't answer.

"Well, we are already on the phone with him switching over care," My husband Leroy said.

"Well, you can't do that, because he told me he can't accept you," she replied.

"Well," we asked, "How do you know that if you said he wasn't answering?" Click. The phone went dead.

We went home, wrote a letter giving the clinic formal notice that we were changing care providers and sent it certified mail.

Since we did switch over care, we didn't think we needed to go to the hospital anymore, and we had also set another appointment with Dr. Bootstaylor for Friday. We headed back to my parents' house, and as I came out of the restroom I saw upset faces and shocked looks on all my family members, who had heard a phone call my husband had just received. He took me by the hands, looked at me and said, "Babe, that was one of my buddies from the Sheriff's department. They are at our apartment with a 'Notice to Apprehend' to deliver you to the hospital for a mandatory psychological evaluation and NST/ultrasound. They said they would give me Officer's courtesy and let us meet them there instead of putting you in the back of the car, but we have to go. Otherwise, they will have to pick you up."

Two deputies escorted us into a different hospital, not the one affiliated with the clinic, and we were met by the Director of Nursing, who had been called in because of this unusual situation. She expressed her negative feelings about what we were being put through. We obviously didn't look like "crazy people" and as we verbalized our predicament, it was good to know we weren't the only ones who thought that something was messed up with this situation. The deputies handed us the notice that the midwife had sent in. It said that I was 48 weeks pregnant! I'm sure that was the overriding reason the judge had signed it. To those of you that are unaware, it is rare to *impossible* for a woman to go 48 weeks, and I certainly wasn't. Sadly, this notice had been looked over and signed by a doctor and a nurse-midwife before it was sent.

After two grueling hours of sitting in a hospital bed, the neonatal specialist was brought into the room and did another NST and ultrasound, and *nothing was wrong*. In fact, everything was the exact same way it had been when we went to the doctor in Atlanta. We had the psychological evaluation, and she said we were being very rational and sensible. We were released without prejudice, but the charges were still in the legal system.

The next morning, my dad was talking to our attorney and he had information that the clinic was not going to drop the charges. We were warned that the next step would be for DFACS to investigate. Since they are considered emergency responders, they could have me forcibly induced. So, in a moderate panic, we packed up the car with suitcases and the home birthing equipment and drove to my aunt's house 4 counties away.

We had a follow-up appointment with Dr. Bootstaylor that Friday, where he told me I was still doing well. After that, we went back to my aunt's house to relax. That evening we attended the book release party for *Baby Designed by God*, and after an awesome party and some pizza, I went into full labor about midnight.

My contractions started a minute apart and went strong for 11 hours, 2 of those full on pushing. We called the doula, Charity, and our parents at 5:30 AM, and they made a fast trip up the highway. I had a normal water home birth. My husband caught our son, calmly unwrapping the cord from his neck with instructions from the doula, with family and friends joining us at that point in the birthing room. Leroy Robert Ward was born at 11:30 AM on November 23rd, 2013, at 9 pounds, 4 ounces and 21 inches long—and *COMPLETELY HEALTHY!*

We would not change any of our decisions, but next time, we could do without all the medical and legal drama. We are thankful for the support of our family, the Drs. Hess, our doula Charity, and Dr. Bootstaylor and his staff.

5.

Woman's Oath of Health

When Susan finally started to connect the pieces about how her health could have been different, how she could have educated herself more about her different health situations, how maybe she could have made better choices, she began to sob uncontrollably. Then she grabbed for the tissues and looked at me straight in the eyes, telling me of all the surgeries and procedures she had over the past 20-plus years and coming to the realization that she couldn't undo many of the decisions she had made about her body. Susan was only 47, and after evaluating the multiple drugs she was taking on a daily basis and her list of surgeries, her words of, *How did my health end up like this?* haunted me for the rest of the day.

As I talked with Jeremy that night about Susan and her medical history, we wondered, how many women are in a similar predicament? How many women fall prey to the possibly unnecessary hysterectomy, the spinal surgery, the cesarean surgical birth, years of antidepressants, cholesterol, blood pressure, thyroid drugs or XYZ treatment, only now to find out that something alternative was never suggested? How many, if they had all the details and information, would have chosen a different path?

Hosea 4:6 reads, "My people are destroyed or perish because of a lack of knowledge." This statement holds true when we view the health of women in this generation. Our soul purpose is to empower women to make educated decisions based on a combination of sound research and exploration of God's design for the female body, in order that they can not only feel good and live well, but also so they can guide and raise up the next generation of women to greater health and awareness.

Like so many of you, over the years I have attempted to make sense of all the constant change in medical opinion, the scientific research, the new pharmaceuticals in the marketplace, and the surgeries and protocols recommended in the face of illness, disease, or other physical affliction. Many times, people confront critical health decisions regarding treatment options and what to do and when—maybe it's chemotherapy, exploratory surgery, or the newest drug to hit the market— any of which could be considered life-changing choices. When facing these unplanned health decisions, we often feel ambushed, caught up in the fear surrounding the issue. I believe that these feelings, along with the sense of "forced" urgency to make a quick decision (whether from well-meaning medical professionals or family members) put people in a state of haste or helplessness. They ignore their intuitive need to take time to pray, weigh options and make an educated decision about their predicament. While I don't question the judgment of the individual doctors or healthcare professionals, I do question the "system" that they operate in. The current "healthcare" system is in serious need of an overhaul.

Let's trace modern medicine to its roots, in hopes of having a better outcome in the future. Hippocrates, the father of medicine, wrote an oath in the late 5th century BC that doctors still adhere to today. The Hippocratic Oath states, "I will prescribe regimens for the good of my patients according to my ability and my judgment and never do harm to anyone."[1] Obviously, doctors aren't intentionally harming their patients, but are they doing harm when their patient is diagnosed with a condition or disease, and the only options presented are pharmaceutical drugs or surgery? Hippocrates, as the father of medicine, also believed in natural methods to promote healing and allow the body to move towards health—not to poison, cover up, kill or "go to war" with our bodies as the current healthcare establishment wants society to believe. My husband and I always say, "Nature or God's creation needs no help; it just needs no interference." Two millennia after Hippocrates came another forward thinker, William Osler, known as the father of modern medicine, and one of the founders of Johns Hopkins University School of Medicine in 1893. He also was a proponent of allowing the body to heal itself with as little intervention as possible. One of my favorite quotations of his many good and common-sense perspectives is, "One of the first duties of the physician is to educate the masses *not* to take medicine."[2] If only our modern doctors would heed his advice and educate the people that drugs should be a final option only

1. "The Hippocratic Oath." National Library of Medicine. http://www.nlm.nih.gov/hmd/greek/greek_oath.html

2. Osler, William. *Sir William Osler: Aphorisms from His Bedside Teachings and Writings.* Ed. Robert Bennett Bean. Henry Schuman, Inc.: New York, 1950. 150.

when all other natural methods have been implemented and given time to work.

A recent Mayo Clinic study found that 70 percent of Americans take at least one prescription drug, over 50 percent of Americans take two prescription drugs, and 20 percent of Americans take five or more drugs![3] And it's not just adults popping pills, either; sadly, in 2007-2008, 20 percent of children reported taking one prescription within the past 30 days. The most commonly prescribed drugs included asthma medications for children, central nervous system stimulants for adolescents, antidepressants for middle-aged adults, and cholesterol-lowering drugs for seniors. In the United States, spending for prescription drugs was $234.1 billion in 2008, which had more than doubled from 1999.[4]

> All women owe it to themselves and their families to view their health as a top priority and not wait until symptoms arise to address their current health situation.

In our practice, we are continually floored by how many pharmaceuticals women say they are taking, as they diligently write them all down on their health history form. Some are on so many, and visit multiple doctors so frequently, that writing it all out would be quite a task; instead, they hand me a medical "resumé" detailing who they visit, what they take, and a year by year list of all the surgeries and/or procedures they have had over their lifetime!

3. "Nearly 7 in 10 Americans Take Prescription Durgs, Mayo Clinic, Olmstead Medical Center Find." Mayo Clinic News Network. http://newsnetwork.mayoclinic.org/discussion/nearly-7-in-10-americans-take-prescription-drugs-mayo-clinic-olmsted-medical-center-find

4. Gu Q, Dillon CF, Burt VL. "Prescription drug use continues to increase: U.S. prescription drug data for 2007-2008." NCHS Data Brief, 42. Hyattsville, MD: National Center for Health Statistics. 2010. http://www.cdc.gov/nchs/data/databriefs/db42.htm

One particularly "popular" group of drugs is the infamously "suspicious" statins or cholesterol drugs. An abundance of research points to the overuse and even misuse of cholesterol-lowering medications. In the US, there are approximately 40 million people currently taking statins to the tune of over $3.00 per pill, costing more than $1,000 per individual per year, totaling more than $40 billion a year.[5] While millions of American adults take statin drugs and are told of all the benefits and wonders of these medications and of artificially lowering your cholesterol, the medical research reveals an untold truth. Multiple studies on statins have shown little to no reason for anyone to take them (with the exception of someone having a previous heart attack), and for women to not take statins for any reason whatsoever![6] As Joseph Mercola, D.O., reports, 99 out of 100 people do not need statin drugs. And even more importantly, cholesterol is not the cause of heart disease.[7] Even though there may be research that contradicts their prescriptions, doctors are caught up adhering to medical protocols and the pharmaceutical industry.

All women owe it to themselves and their families to view their health as a top priority and not wait until symptoms arise to address their current health situation. Recently, a close friend of mine discovered that at the young age of 56, her mother had just been diagnosed with breast cancer. Although she plans on supporting her mother in whichever route of treatment she

5. Carey, John. "Do Cholesterol Drugs Do Any Good?" *Bloomberg Businessweek Magazine.* http://www.businessweek.com/stories/2008-01-16/do-cholesterol-drugs-do-any-good

6. Topol, Eric J. "The Diabetes Dilemma for Statin Users." *The New York Times* March 4, 2012. http://www.nytimes.com/2012/03/05/opinion/the-diabetes-dilemma-for-statin-users.html?_r=0

7. Mercola, Joseph. "The Cholesterol Myth That Could Be Harming Your Health." *Huffington Post* August 12, 2010. http://www.huffingtonpost.com/dr-mercola/the-cholesterol-myth-that_b_676817.html

consents to having (which is most likely to be the traditional medical model of radiation, chemotherapy, and/or mastectomy), she confided that her mother has neglected her health for years and is now facing a life-threatening situation. For many years, she has urged her mother to seek out natural health providers and change her lifestyle habits; however, her mother and many of her close family members make fun of her for her "natural" lifestyle. My friend told me that her mother is approximately 50 pounds overweight, loves to eat sugar-infested sweets, regularly drinks soda and other beverages full of artificial sweeteners and chemicals, hasn't exercised on a regular basis in years, frequents fast food establishments, refuses to buy natural home and personal care products, and is basically living like the average American, who waits until a health crisis occurs to take action and attempt lifestyle changes. The recent diagnosis of breast cancer—even though she followed her doctor's recommendations of routine mammograms over the years—is a repeated story heard too often. We pray for her mother's healing, but are left with this question: Would she be in this health crisis had she made better health and lifestyle choices for herself?

What makes sense to me is the natural and conservative health approach first, which begins with prevention, so we encounter these situations far less often.

Everyone can agree that all pharmaceuticals and surgeries have minor to serious side effects. Our mothers, sisters, daughters, friends and even we ourselves face serious illnesses of all kinds, but there are many natural solutions and options to help the body heal itself without having to resort to toxic pharmaceuticals or dangerous surgeries. What makes sense to me is the natural and conservative health approach first, which begins with prevention, so we encounter these situations far less often. Yes, drugs or surgery can serve as a last resort, but should they be the first option? In obvious emergency or crisis-care situations, pharmaceuticals and surgeries may save lives, but emergency care accounts for a very small percentage of the overall healthcare system. The real issue that we are facing as a society is that instead of people taking care of themselves on a regular basis, they are taught to wait for symptoms to show up before they do anything proactive for their bodies or health. If we have no "symptoms," we are thought to be healthy. Only when we manifest symptoms do we think that we are "sick" or "something is wrong." The modern "healthcare" model then takes over by covering up the symptom with a drug, and when that doesn't work, then they can just cut it out.

What would happen if women were taught to eat whole, organic foods, practice routine exercise, supplement on a daily basis with nutritionally supportive vitamins, minerals and herbs, receive regular specific chiropractic care, use organic cosmetic and household products, and utilize natural methods of living? I believe we would have a health revolution, and women would live their lives in better health the way God intended. I believe that God created the body to heal from the inside out. God gave us specific, inborn bodily systems, like a properly functioning nervous system and an immune system that knows exactly how to purge itself of toxins or fight an infection. I also believe God gave us natural methods of healing, like chiropractic, whole foods from the earth, naturopathy, herbology, and so many other wonderful, safe, useful and effective methods that work with the innate healing potential of our bodies to promote health and longevity.

In today's modern system of "healthcare," the Hippocratic Oath can only go so far. What if there was a new kind of oath, one that emphasized personal responsibility, one that all women would vow and honor? We've put it on a page by itself so that you can cut it out, sign and display it on your fridge, mirror, or somewhere else in your home/work to remind you of your commitment to healthy living designed by God.

Woman's Oath of Health

As a woman, a wife, a mother, a sister, a grandmother,
viewing my body as a temple of the Holy Spirit,

I solemnly promise that I will, to the best of my ability, make
wise health choices on a daily basis.

I recognize that the role of a woman has considerable
responsibility, and I will not abuse nor neglect my health and
wait for a health crisis to occur.

I will seek out natural organic foods, cosmetics, household
products and naturally-minded healthcare professionals for
my family and myself.

I will educate myself and surround myself with like-minded,
health-conscious individuals.

I will question possibly unnecessary procedures and protocols
before I consent to standard medical systems for my family or
myself.

I will recognize the limits of my knowledge and seek to
increase God-given health principles throughout my life.

I make this declaration solemnly, freely and upon my honor.

Signature:_____

Live a Natural, Holistic Life Based on God's Design

Inspired by *Woman Designed by God*

Jennifer Gore

Let me start off by saying that I am so thankful for Drs. Jeremy and Amanda Hess. My life is forever changed because of these two amazing individuals. They have loved me, prayed for me, adjusted me, educated me and given me the opportunity of a lifetime, and for that I am forever grateful.

I would like to go back to the beginning to help you understand the health struggles I have been through. To start things off, I was born a month early. My mom was given a "twilight shot" to ease her pain. I was supposed to be a breech baby, but I decided to flip at the last minute. I was born with reflux, yellow jaundice, a weak immune system and digestion problems, and I was on a heart monitor because I would stop breathing from time to time. Also, because my mom had milk fever, she was told not to breastfeed me. By the time I was 3 months old, I had several doctors and had spent weeks at Scottish Rite Hospital. I was receiving a lot of medical treatments, along with more medication than a child should probably be taking at that age.

As I got older, my health only got worse. From the time I was born until I turned 2 years old, I was only able to have sugar water and rice water. Between the ages of 3 and 18 years old, I had severe allergies, nose bleeds, sinus problems, constant ear infections, chronic strep throat, Irritable Bowel Syndrome, 5 cases of chicken pox, shingles, scarlet fever and German measles (even though I was vaccinated as a child). I had horrible menstrual cycles, scoliosis and migraine headaches that started at age 13. When I was 18, I had my tonsils and adenoids removed, hoping it would help, but it didn't. I missed 32 days of school my senior year due to my health.

At the age of 18, I was rear ended in a car accident. I had some pain but thought I was young and it would go away on its own. At 19 I was rear ended again, and this time it was much worse. I was in a lot of pain and went to the hospital, where I received lots of pain medication, and later I was sent to an orthopedist, who put me in physical therapy for 6 weeks. After the accident, I noticed my headaches getting worse and more frequent, so I went to a neurologist. After the neurologist did a MRI, CAT scan, EMG, and sleep study, I was diagnosed with narcolepsy, as well as a brain tumor on my hypothalamus gland. I was given many different medications for migraine headaches, and I was given Adderall for the narcolepsy. I was told I would take these medications the rest of my life if I wanted to be able to function and drive a car.

A few years later, when I was 21, I was rear ended for the third time. This accident was the straw that broke the camel's back. I was having severe pain in my lower back, left hip, and down my left leg into my foot. My left foot stayed numb all the time, and I could barely walk. I couldn't really sit or stand, and my mom had to help dress me, bathe me and assist me in going to the bathroom. I was sent to another orthopedist that decided to treat me with 3 epidurals and pain pills. The doctor also performed 2 nerve conduction studies and a discogram, and he sent me to physical therapy 3 times per week for 8 months, had me getting acupuncture, and put me on a TENS unit (an electric nerve stimulator). After 8 months of physical therapy, I was not any better, so my doctors wrote letters to another physical therapist, who was considered to be the best of the best. The doctors begged him to see me and after several attempts he finally accepted me. He specialized more in nerves and less on muscles, but after a few months, he was also unable to help me.

I was then sent to a neurosurgeon, who performed a myelogram. After finding nothing, he sent me back to the orthopedist. The orthopedist said my test showed damaged nerves and discs, but my MRI looked almost perfect. He said that at that point, he was diagnosing me with plantar fasciitis, sciatica and degenerative disc disease. He then suggested trying a new procedure that he had never done before, and I would be his "guinea pig." I didn't like the sound of that, so I asked him about my other options. He decided that he wanted to perform exploratory back surgery. At the same time, my neurologist suggested having brain surgery to remove the tumor, but I only had a 20 percent chance of living through the surgery. I was also warned that if I lived through the surgery that I would have to re-learn some major motor skills i.e. how to walk, talk, write, etc. But the good news was that I wouldn't have migraine headaches anymore, and my narcolepsy would go away as well.

On top of all these decisions to make at the age of 23, I was having horrible menstrual cycles. My OBGYN advised me that she thought I either had endometriosis or PCOS (polycystic ovarian syndrome), but she would need to scrape and clip some tissue to run some tests. I declined both tests. I was also told that I had a tilted uterus and would never be able to conceive, and if I ever conceived I would miscarry. The OBGYN advised me that since cancer runs in my family, it might be a good idea to have a hysterectomy. I had a lot of life-changing decisions to make at a very young age. I remember telling the orthopedist that I would pray about my decision, and he got a grin on his face and said to me, "Where has that gotten you so far?" I was appalled that he would even say such a thing to me. I then asked him about going to a chiropractor. He immediately said, "Do not go to a chiropractor, because if you do, they will paralyze you."

At that point, I felt lost and confused. I was hopeless and couldn't see the light at the end of the tunnel. I was 23 years of age taking 24 prescription drugs daily. Here are just a few of them: Lortab, Darvocet, Flexeril, Imitrex, 2 birth controls (because my cycles were so bad), Wellbutrin (which caused me to have seizures), Adderall, Claritin, and the list goes on and on. Each medication carried side effects, which led to more health problems. I decided to pray about my decisions and put my life in God's hands. In March of 2010, I found an ad in a local shopper paper with information about Discover Chiropractic. The ad talked about the technology they used and testimonies from people about their healing. I figured I had tried everything else; why not try this too? So, I called and made an appointment. That appointment changed my life forever.

I remember coming to the office and the ladies there being so loving and understanding. I also remember attending the new patient class. This is a time where the doctors take time out of their schedule to explain what they do and why they do what they do. I remember hearing the doctors speak and thinking to myself, *Wow, they are telling my story—they are talking about me*. But the memory that stands out the most is the first time I met Dr. Jeremy Hess. I remember saying to him, "I don't trust you. You have to earn my trust. Every doctor told me they could help me, and they didn't. I am only giving you 3 adjustments, and if I am not feeling better I will not be back." He looked at me, smiled and responded, "You have a lot going on, but we are going to help you. My job is to put everything back in place, and God will heal your body. Now let's pray together." That prayer made all the difference in the world. Finally, there was someone who cared about me!

Dr. Hess was the first doctor to check my neck and not just my back. After the first adjustment, I was able to walk on my own and sit normally. By my second adjustment, I was able to go a couple of days without pain medication. And by my third adjustment, I was able to stick my foot in the bathtub and feel the temperature of the water for the first time in over a year. Since I am a person who believes in keeping my word, I continued my care after those 3 adjustments, and that was one of the best decisions I have ever made. Within a year, I was off all of my medications except for the Adderall, which took longer to wean off. I began eating less processed food, eating more organic options and less gluten. I traded in the harsh, chemically laden chemicals and cosmetics around my house for more natural products. My daily pill intake went from cover-up-the-symptom pharmaceuticals to life-giving vitamins. I also was able to begin exercising for the first time in many years.

Growing up, I always thought health came from a pharmacy. My parents didn't know any differently, so I didn't know any differently. As I got older, if I could find a pill or cream to fix something, I would take it. As a Christian I understood that God made my body, but never understood how He designed it to function. I finally have the knowledge to understand better. I truly believe that if people knew what I know, they would do what I do, and that's why I try to educate people everyday. I am 100 percent prescription drug free and haven't been to a medical doctor in almost 4 years.

But the biggest news in my life is that I have a beautiful 4-month-old little girl. When I found out I was pregnant, I decided to hire a midwife and have a natural birth. I understood that God made my body to give birth, and He gave me this blessing to protect. I received chiropractic care during my entire pregnancy. I chose to only have one ultrasound when I was pregnant, so we didn't really know how big she was, but we knew that God made her to fit perfectly in my body so I wasn't worried about her coming out. On October 21, 2013, my water broke. After getting to the hospital and being in labor for a few hours, my midwife discovered that our baby girl was face up with her head tilted back. They call this an OP baby, and according to the medical model, OP babies are suppose to be taken out by C-section. But not our little girl! My husband was my doula and was super supportive. While I was in labor, he kept me calm and kept reminding me about how God designed my body to give birth. I wouldn't have been able to do it without him; he was my strength and my rock through the whole birth. After 18 hours of labor (2 hours of pushing), I gave birth to a beautiful, 9 pound, 4 ounces, 22-inch-long baby girl! After giving birth to Ryleigh, I made a promise to

God that I would protect her and love her with every ounce of my body. I also made a promise to Ryleigh that I would never inject her with anything that I wouldn't put in a cup and let her drink. She got her first chiropractic adjustment at 24 hours old. She is not vaccinated, and she is breastfed. At 4 months old, she hasn't been sick at all.

I am thankful for what I now know so that I can be a better mom and give my daughter the life that God has designed for her to have. I am so thankful that Drs. Jeremy and Amanda Hess educated my family and me. It is a great feeling knowing that you have a support system that believes in you and supports your decisions. My hope and prayer is that if you are reading this, you now have more hope than you had before. There is light at the end of the tunnel, and you deserve to have the life God designed for you to have.

6.

Sweet Curves

"I love all kinds of bread. Whenever I crave junk food,
I want salty things like peanuts or potato chips."
– Tyra Banks

"I love to eat—Kit Kats or cookies-and-cream ice
cream. I need sugar like five times a day."
– Kim Kardashian

"My food demons are Chinese food, sugar, butter."
– Kirstie Alley

"The best part of any meal is dessert. Preferably a
dessert with chocolate."
– Dr. Amanda Hess

We love to laugh at what people say about food and how they are starting their "diet" on Monday or after the next upcoming vacation. Just like everyone else, we battle sugar, processed foods and our food intake every day, at every meal, and when we shop at the grocery store or eat out away from the home. One of our goals is to not bring too many sugars or processed foods into the home. That way, neither we or the kids will even be tempted to eat our "food demons." Now, this is not to say the kids don't talk us into a stop at Yoforia, one of their favorite organic yogurt shops in Atlanta, nor does Jeremy never persuade me to buy chocolate for him at our favorite chocolatier every once in a while. We all have the freedom to eat what we want, while having the knowledge of what is good and bad for us. One thing we always say is, "If it's in the house, it'll end up in your belly," thereby messing with any and all health goals you have set for yourself or the family to eat consistently healthy, keep the extra pounds off and avoid chronic disease and illness. You can still have the freedom to eat different things, just as long as you're *consistently consuming* foods that are wholesome and good for you.

> You can still have the freedom to eat different things, just as long as you're *consistently* consuming foods that are wholesome and good for you.

I remember about five years ago, the practice was busy, our family life with a new baby now had sped up a bit, and we were also moving our chiropractic practice to a new location, so Jeremy was eating more on the run. Now, when I say on the run, most people might automatically assume that means a drive-through fast food chain. Well, with Jeremy typically always moving at 80 miles an hour anyways, this actually meant that he had shifted to start including Starbucks lattés and Frappuccinos, green smoothie drinks and other carbohydrates like chips, crackers and crunchy grains into his diet. The carbs he was eating were mostly organic, whole food and from good sources, but they were still carbs, which translate into sugars and in many cases manifest as fat. Because Jeremy is always going at Mach 2 speed, he never got fat; he just started suffering with symptoms of too many sugars and grains. The "healthy" green smoothie drinks contained lots of good stuff like spirulina, wheat grass, and fruits, but they were loaded with sugar…albeit naturally occurring sugar. In fact, one bottle of the "healthy green juice" contained a whopping 56 grams of sugar, not far off from a 16-ounce, blended caramel coffee drink, which contains 64 grams! After about six months of this, I remember he started complaining about feeling bloated, sluggish, and even unexplainably moody. What Jeremy was really experiencing was gut imbalance, very typical of the average American who is eating lots of grain-based carbohydrates and eating or drinking tons of sugar.

Today, the average American consumes almost 152 pounds of sugar in one year; in comparison, two hundred years ago, the average American ate only two pounds of sugar a year.[1, 2] Many people don't realize that this excessive sugar intake can contribute to a weakened immune system and a myriad of other diseases. In our other book, *Baby Designed by God*, we discuss how so many children get sick and immune-compromised around Halloween and other sugar-intensive holidays, and how sugar and carbohydrates are "king" at daycares and schools. Some current research studies also are pointing the finger at sugar as a contributing factor in cancer growth. Obviously,

1. USDA. *Agriculture Fact Book 2001-2002.* United States Department of Agriculture. http://www.usda.gov/documents/usda-factbook-2001-2002.pdf

2. New Hampshire Department of Health and Human Services. "How Much Sugar Do You Eat? You May Be Surprised!" DHHS. http://www.dhhs.state.nh.us/dphs/nhp/adults/documents/sugar.pdf

further studies are warranted, but the following highlights one small study involving mice and breast tumors:

> *A mouse model of human breast cancer demonstrated that tumors are sensitive to blood-glucose levels. Sixty-eight mice were injected with an aggressive strain of breast cancer, and then fed diets to induce high blood sugar (hyperglycemia), normoglycemia or low blood sugar (hypoglycemia).* **There was a dose-dependent response in which the lower the blood glucose, the greater the survival rate.** *After 70 days, 8 of 24 hyperglycemic mice survived, compared to 16 of 24 normoglycemic and 19 of 20 hypoglycemic. This suggests that regulating sugar intake is key to slowing breast tumor growth.*[3]

Although major medical studies don't say outright that sugar causes cancer, Clare McKindley, clinical dietitian at MD Anderson's Cancer Prevention Center, states, "But too much daily sugar can cause weight gain. And, unhealthy weight gain and a lack of exercise can increase your cancer risks."[4] In fact, the American Heart Association states that women should have no more than six teaspoons of sugar per day (25 grams), and men should have no more than nine teaspoons per day (37 grams).[5] These guidelines are virtually impossible for the

3. Quillin, Patrick. "Cancer's Sweet Tooth." Mercola. http://www.mercola.com/article/sugar/sugar_cancer.htm

4. Espat, Adelina. "Does cancer love sugar?" *Focused on Health* November 2012. http://www.mdanderson.org/publications/focused-on-health/issues/2012-november/cancersugar.html

5. American Heart Association. "Sugar 101." AHA. http://www.heart.org/HEARTORG/Getting-Healthy/NutritionCenter/HealthyEating/Sugar-101_UCM_306024_Article.jsp

How Much Sugar Is in *Your* Favorite Drink?

Huge quantities of sugar lurk in some common popular beverages. How many of these do you consume every day? Every week? Note that just one of these drinks far exceeds the recommended daily amount of sugar for women!

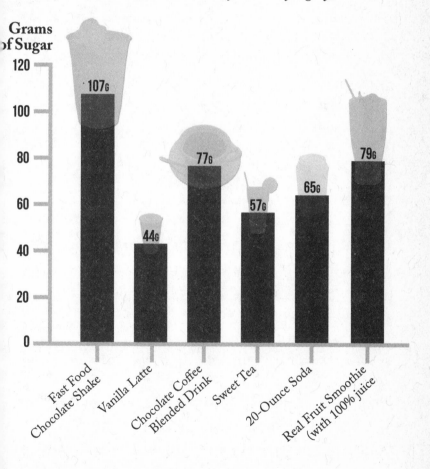

Grams of Sugar

Fast Food Chocolate Shake	107ɢ
Vanilla Latte	44ɢ
Chocolate Coffee Blended Drink	77ɢ
Sweet Tea	57ɢ
20-Ounce Soda	65ɢ
Real Fruit Smoothie (with 100% juice)	79ɢ

Calculations based on large-sized beverages from popular national fast food chains.

average American to abide by when one 12-ounce can of Coke contains 39 grams of sugar.

Some readers may think that this news about sugar is no big deal, because they eat and drink items that are deemed "sugar-free." What this label really means, however, is that these consumables contain artificial sweeteners. Yes, there are some studies out there indicating a link between artificial sweeteners and cancer, but the scientific community still won't say that there is enough proof. I am always floored by the overweight men and women who are always sipping on their "diet" soft drinks. It's like they think they are making a healthy choice, but until more studies have been done, everyone should avoid or limit artificial sweeteners as much as possible.

So, how much is too much sugar?

Most Americans are oblivious to the fact that with every sip or bite they take of sugary foods, they are not only adding inches to their waistline, but are also slowly damaging themselves. Right around the corner from our practice are two of Atlanta's most iconic fast food establishments that reign in our area as "the places to go." One serves a very popular milkshake that hails at over 100 grams of sugar in a large; the other serves up sweet iced tea ranging in sugar content from 60 to 119 grams per serving.[6, 7] It's no wonder why conditions like heart disease, digestive disorders, cancer, diabetes and obesity are such a problem with so many of us.

---

6. Chick-Fil-A Nutrition Facts. http://www.chick-fil-a.com/Food/Menu-Detail/Strawberry-Milkshake# ?details=nutrition&variation=strawberrylarge

7. Krispy Kreme Donuts Nutritional Information. http://www.krispykreme.com/SharedContent/Media/NutritionalLibrary/Nutritional_Template_01142013.pdf

So how much is too much sugar? This is exactly what Jeremy starting looking at when he started getting symptomatic with his sugar overloads. "Added sugar" is exactly that: added sugars found mainly in processed foods, *not* the sugar found naturally in foods like fruits and vegetables. Once he stopped his sugar highs and constant carbs and switched over to water, protein, vegetables and some fruit, he lost 15 pounds in less than a month. We always joke about his weight loss because people who haven't seen him in a long time always comment about how thin he is now. Even going through airport security, we laugh because the TSA agents will look at his driver's license, do a double take and exclaim, "Wow, you've lost weight!"

In January, I was just finishing up a chiropractic adjustment on a woman, when she stopped me before I had left the room. "Dr. Amanda," she said, "how do you stay so slim? What's your secret?" This conversation led to a discussion of what she was eating and the changes she had been making for the last few months, such as eating better and trying to lose weight. She started to tell me how she had switched to whole grains and brown rice, organic breads, flour and pasta. Even the snacks she was buying now were "organic and GMO-free." I applauded her efforts, as Jeremy and I will go out of our way to shop at grocery stores and frequent restaurants that utilize organic and GMO-free options.

I went on to explain to her about sugars and carbohydrates. Our bodies process excessive carbohydrate intake, and unless you are an extreme athlete and burning off the excess, then in most cases you will retain or continue to gain weight. I clarified that using organic and GMO-free items is a must, and that they were a good choice and worthwhile investment, but she was still eating too many grains and carbohydrates as her main intake of food, which is why she couldn't shed the pounds. I suggested to her a specific approach to follow, eating protein, vegetables, and some fruit while eliminating or limiting breads, pastas and boxed snacks. It would also be a good idea to limit or totally eliminate dairy and gluten, and of course, drink lots of water (saying goodbye to Southern sweet tea and soft drinks). She said she would look into my recommendations. Two weeks later, she came back for another chiropractic adjustment at the office and said she was "jumping all in" with my recommendations. I high-fived and encouraged her, and within a month, she had lost 19 pounds!

Some of you reading might relate to a good friend of mine, who feels like she has tried everything and can't take the weight off. Unfortunately for her and so many other women, they have no idea about one big problem our industrialized society has caused us. Yes, it has given us all kinds of good things like hair dryers, cell phones, Tupperware, any type of food whenever we want it, and the chance to travel to exotic destinations, but in the process, technology has created something called *xenoestrogens*. What are those and how do you even pronounce the word? I thought the same thing during my research when I first came across the term. It's a term you should become familiar with, as these are causing chronic illness and weight gain in many women. Xenoestrogens are a type of faux-hormone that imitates estrogen. They can take the form of either synthetic or natural chemical compounds.

Beginner's Guide to
Avoiding Xenoestrogens

STEER CLEAR OF

Caffeine

Commercial dairy products

Reheating/consuming foods
in plastic or Styrofoam
containers

Commercially-raised, non-organic
meats and poultry

Household/personal
products containing
phosphates, parabens,
or phthalates

Unfiltered water
(water you drink and
water you bathe in)

Industrial chemicals found
in commercial sunscreens,
food preservatives, insecticides,
pesticides, herbicides, etc.

Oral contraceptives,
synthetic hormone
replacement therapies,
chlorinated/chemically laden
tampons and sanitary napkins

Bleached coffee filters

HERE ARE SOME THINGS THAT YOU CAN DO

- USE glass or ceramic containers to store food and water

- AVOID plastics and especially heating plastics in the microwave

- REPLACE your laundry, dish and household cleaners with natural alternatives

- BUY organic meat, poultry, produce and dairy products

- REPLACE your cosmetic and skincare products

- INVEST in a water filtration system for the entire home

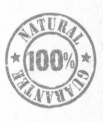

For those readers who are in menopause (or know someone who is), many of you face hormone imbalance and issues of estrogen dominance, which causes challenges regarding weight and fat retention. Too much estrogen in your body can make you gain weight, and at a fast pace! Excess estrogen in your body increases body fat, and in turn, fatty tissue in your body will produce more estrogen. You can see how the two feed off each other and ultimately cause you to gain more weight and increase your waistline. Interestingly, though, estrogen dominance is not caused by menopause alone. In our industrialized society, we continually encounter xenoestrogens, which pass into our bodies through all kinds of environmental exposure, in things like pesticides, herbicides and fungicides on many of our foods and clothing, as well as common use of plastics and cosmetics, exposure to car exhausts, dry cleaning chemicals, industrial waste, hormones in our meat, poultry and food, and countless other household and personal products which many of us use everyday.[8]

Since the problem of xenoestrogens has been growing more rampant in our society in recent years, many in the health community believe that the spike in younger women with PMS, fibrocystic breast disease, PCOS, infertility, endometriosis, mood swings, and issues with weight gain is strongly related. In fact, about three months ago, I was talking with a natural health provider about infertility. I told her that in many cases, chiropractic adjustments can help by correcting nerve interference caused by misalignments in the lower back and pelvic areas of the spine, as those nerves are related to

8. Miller, Magnolia. "What Are Xenoestrogens and How Do They Make You Fat?" Healthline. http://www.healthline.com/health-blogs/hold-that-pause/what-are-xenoestrogens-fat

female reproductive function. She then began to tell me of three women she had helped in the last year, all between the ages of 25 and 35, who were having trouble with infertility. As she consulted with each of them, she pinpointed that a common denominator between them was the consumption of high amounts of hormones in the poultry and meat they were eating. As each of them made dietary changes to organic foods, with an emphasis on eating only organic poultry and meats, all three were able to become pregnant within the next ten months!

On page 89, you will find a short beginner's guide on how to avoid as many xenoestrogens as possible.

I believe that most women are willing to make changes, but because of so much misinformation on health topics, many women end up hopeless, not knowing whom to trust, which way to turn or what to do. My prayer and hope is that this book will provide hope and clarity for every woman's health journey, as I know and believe God designed our bodies for optimal health and wants us to fulfill His purpose on this earth, and it can be achieved only when our bodies are functioning at their highest God-given potential.

My Natural Weight Loss Story

By Herta Thomas and Meri Warbrick, Naturopath

I have struggled with my weight for many years—losing 20 pounds, regaining 25, losing 25, and regaining 30. You know the story, especially those of you struggling with your own weight issues.

Allow me to share my success story and what prompted me to lose weight for the final time. My most recent weight loss was prompted by an upcoming visit to Germany. I was excited about the trip, but I was 40 pounds overweight and I had a few health issues: poor digestion, a bad knee, and abdominal pain. My family was concerned because I was reluctant to see a medical doctor; however, after many weeks of discomfort, I decided my family was right. I should check things out—after all, insurance would cover it, right?

So began my medical journey. Because of my symptoms, the gastroentrologist felt we should start with an endoscopy and a colonoscopy. When the tests were completed and the results were back, the diagnosis was nothing definite, with only a little redness. Now that was hard to believe. All my discomfort was from possible Irritable Bowel Syndrome (IBS) and a little redness? Nothing found! Yet I was not to escape so easily, for the doctor felt my symptoms could be improved with several prescriptions (wait until you hear this experience). I was given Omeprazole to reduce the acid in my stomach and to treat symptoms of reflux. This gave me nausea. For the nausea, I received Promethazine. Dicyclomine was given to control pain caused by IBS. This caused me to have bloating, nausea, and constipation. To combat the constipation I received Amitiza, resulting in water retention. Finally I decided, *Enough meds! They are trying to kill me!*

The next phase of my story is so much more exciting. I decided to seek out natural solutions, as the myriad of pharmaceuticals was taking its toll on me. My friend and naturopath, Meri, had encouraged me to check things out with my physician to satisfy my family and to make me feel more comfortable with the natural route. Once I knew there was nothing seriously wrong with me, I was ready to begin. First on my list was weight loss. I would be seeing friends and family on my aforementioned trip to Germany, and I wanted to dazzle them with a slimmer me.

Are you ready? Here's the plan and the results. My first step was a 21-day purification regimen. This time I was committed and followed my regime 100 percent. I didn't cheat! Yeah! The results were astonishing. I was 18 pounds lighter after those three short weeks. *Get ready, Germany, here I come.* I was concerned about being away and not being able to control my diet, but guess what? I lost another three pounds while I was in Germany visiting with friends and family. Five weeks later, I was back home and continuing my weight loss. How could I continue to lose the additional 22 pounds that I had set as my goal?

My Naturopath had been encouraging me to give up grains and dairy; she felt it would improve my few remaining health symptoms. My new weight loss plan: breakfast included nutritional enhancing shakes with almond milk and three different spices; lunch was a huge salad with vegetables and four ounces of protein, and coconut oil with spices as my choice for a salad dressing; dinner was four ounces of protein with more steamed vegetables. I also added 32 ounces of lemon water first thing in the morning, followed later in the day by 32 ounces of water with apple cider vinegar, followed still later by an additional 32 ounces of water, for a total of 96 ounces of water daily.

Let me share my total results! I am now 43 pounds lighter and my thighs are no longer 27 inches…they are 21 inches. And my knee pain is gone along with my 27-inch thighs! I spent years dreaming of beautiful, slim thighs, and now I have them. Now how is that for success? My health is excellent, too—no more stomach problems. My daily food choices still consist of mainly protein, vegetables, a small amount of fruit, nutritional shakes, and a lot of water. I do occasionally splurge and have a healthy sweet snack. I have attempted to reintroduce small amounts of grains and dairy into my diet, but because of their negative effects on my digestive system, I have eliminated both from my diet.

Posted below are my before and after pictures. If I can achieve success naturally, so can YOU!

Before

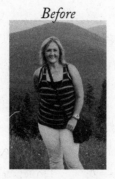

After

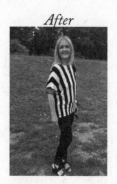

7.

That Time of the Month

Aunt Flo is visiting. My monthly visitor is back. The crimson tide has returned. The monthly menstrual cycle. It happens to all of us, that unknown time of the month when we have to be extra cautious of what we wear and about our feminine hygiene. Every woman remembers when and where it first happened to us. Some of us were anxiously awaiting the moment of "officially" becoming a woman, and others of us might have felt like it was our own little atomic bomb event. Either way, we got through it.

I remember being in high school with all my other girlfriends who were already developing and having their menstrual cycle. I was the last one to get it, almost believing that I was just some sort of tall, skinny, flat-chested, toothpick-legged girl who would never step into womanhood. No one ever gave me a lecture on my menstrual cycle or even explained feminine hygiene products to me. I basically learned from watching my mother and older sister go through the monthly process of having their cycle, and by default I knew to look under the bathroom cabinets and start studying the side of the box to see how to use tampons and maxi pads correctly.

As a mother with young kids, it is a rare occasion to actually be able to go to the bathroom alone; hence, my own daughter Alyssa, who is 7 years old, has already begun asking questions about why Mommy sometimes bleeds down there. Since she is only 7, I felt like I had a number of years ahead of me before I really needed to approach the topic. Then, I began to notice other boys and girls her age or a little older showing signs of precocious puberty. Some girls as young as 8 are starting to menstruate, develop breasts and grow pubic and underarm hair—all of which are secondary sex characteristics. In decades past, these "biological milestones" typically occurred only at age 13 or older.[1] However, the age of menarche (the first occurrence of menstruation) has been consistently decreasing over the past 100 years. A new study published in *Pediatrics* measured the proportion of girls who had entered puberty by ages 7 and 8, and saw striking increases compared to data collected in 1997, only 13 years ago. This study of US girls found that by age 7, 10.4 percent of Caucasian girls (up from 5 percent in 1997), 23.4 percent of African-American girls (15 percent in 1997), and 14.9 percent of Hispanic girls had already entered puberty. By age 8, the percentages had reached 18.3 percent, 42.9 percent, and 30.9 percent, respectively.[2]

As I studied further, I didn't like what I learned, as research also indicates that girls who experience early puberty carry a well-established risk factor for breast cancer later in life.[3] And

1. Steingraber, Sandra. "The Falling Age of Puberty in U.S. Girls: What We Know, What We Need to Know." Breast Cancer Fund. http://www.breastcancerfund.org/assets/pdfs/publications/falling-age-of-puberty-adv-guide.pdf

2. Biro FM, Galvez MP, Greenspan LC, et al. "Pubertal Assessment Method and Baseline Characteristics in a Mixed Longitudinal Study of Girls." *Pediatrics* September 2010, 126(3), 583-90. http://pediatrics.aappublications.org/content/early/2010/08/09/peds.2009-3079.full.pdf+html

3. Vandeloo MJ, Bruckers LM, Janssens JP. "Effects of lifestyle on the onset of puberty as determinant for breast cancer." *European Journal of Cancer Prevention*, February 2007, 16(1),17-25.

by the way, ladies, if you have a son or grandson, early onset of puberty for boys is associated with increased rates of prostate and testicular cancer later in life.[4] So what's causing this early onset of puberty? Research is finding that the main causes of early onset of puberty is obesity in childhood ages from 3 to 7 years old, as this increases a girl's exposure to estrogen.

Most of the research also points to excess consumption of animal proteins at an early age. The commentaries don't say never to eat meat or other animal proteins; they merely suggest that most kids are eating too much of the common "Western" diet of meat, cheese, and processed foods, with many parents just not knowing it can cause so much harm. A 2010 study found that girls with the highest meat intake at age 7 were 75 percent more likely to have begun menstruating by age 12½ than those in the lowest category of meat intake.[5] Some speculation has been raised over the increased use of hormones in the foods many children eat on a regular basis.[6]

This is one reason we've shifted our budget and spend less money on things like clothing and technology items, instead placing more value on what type of foods we buy. We recommend you do the same for yourselves and your family. Along with getting routine chiropractic care to keep the nervous system, the master controller of the body, functioning at optimal levels, we believe strongly in the huge impact that eating organic,

4. Günther AL, et al. "Dietary protein intake throughout childhood is associated with the timing of puberty." *Journal of Nutrition*, March 2010, 140(3):565-71. http://jn.nutrition.org/content/140/3/565.full

5. Fuhrman, Joel. "Girls are reaching puberty earlier than ever." Disease Proof. http://www.diseaseproof.com/archives/cat-girls.html

6. "Girls are Reaching Puberty Earlier Than Ever." https://www.drfuhrman.com/library/early_puberty.aspx

natural and whole foods can make on your overall long term health.

Once our sons and daughters do reach puberty, hopefully at a more mature age than 7 or 8 years old, we need to start educating them on how their bodies work and what God designed them for—to be holy and used for His glory. The subject of sex must be addressed, and it's necessary to teach them our beliefs and what is right and acceptable. Crucial in this conversation obviously is the topic of abstinence, so I want to discuss my issues with birth control pills (or related hormone-regulating medications) from the perspective of adolescent girls or women using it as a means of regulating their periods, or simply using them for contraception. Now, keep in mind, many young girls and teenagers, as well as many older women, are being prescribed birth control before they are married, for reasons other than "contraception."

> The subject of sex must be addressed, and it's necessary to teach children our beliefs and what is right and acceptable.

Research finds that more than half (58 percent) of all birth control pill users rely on the method, at least in part, for purposes other than pregnancy prevention. One study, based on US government data from the National Survey of Family Growth (NSFG), revealed that after pregnancy prevention (86 percent), the most common reasons women use the Pill include reducing cramps or menstrual pain (31 percent); menstrual regulation, which for some women may help prevent migraines and other painful "side effects" of menstruation (28 percent); treatment of acne (14 percent); and treatment of endometriosis (4 percent). Additionally, the study

Risks of the Pill

Research finds that that more than half (**58%**) of all birth control pill users rely on the method, at least in part, for purposes other than pregnancy prevention.

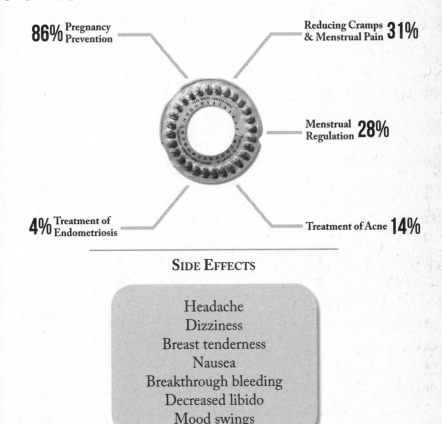

86% Pregnancy Prevention

Reducing Cramps & Menstrual Pain **31%**

Menstrual Regulation **28%**

4% Treatment of Endometriosis

Treatment of Acne **14%**

SIDE EFFECTS

Headache
Dizziness
Breast tenderness
Nausea
Breakthrough bleeding
Decreased libido
Mood swings

Bryner, Jeanna. "Many Teens Rely on the Pill for Non-Sexual Reasons." LiveScience. November 26, 2011. http://www.livescience.com/17061-oral-contraceptive-pill-guttmacher-survey.html

Health.com, "7 Common Birth Control Side Effects." http://www.health.com/health/gallery/0,,20408202_2,00.html

found that some 762,000 women who have never had sex use the Pill, and they do so almost exclusively (99 percent) for non-contraceptive reasons.[7] So what's so wrong with women trying ease their migraines, acne or other related female symptoms? The problem arises when we artificially alter our hormones in the body (whether it be short-term or long-term), as it may cause health effects in our future.

The Pill contains two synthetic hormones (progestin and ethinyl estradiol) and has three mechanisms: 1) it prevents ovulation, 2) thickens the cervical mucus, which makes it harder for sperm to enter the uterus and 3) affects the endometrium, or lining of the uterus, to make it more hostile to implantation. Maybe it's just me, but I can't imagine it's good to "prevent ovulation" long-term and intentionally interfere with the body's normal physiological mechanisms.

Furthermore, how could it be morally acceptable to prevent implantation? This means that the egg and sperm *did* meet, unite and begin the trek over to implantation, but now we have artificially altered the uterine lining so the embryo cannot attach and thus dies—essentially, a very early abortion. Some forms of birth control methods offer a "fake menstrual cycle" of withdrawal bleeding (which makes women believe they are having a "normal" menstrual cycle), while other forms may offer withdrawal bleeding only four times per year. Some women choose to suppress their menstrual cycle altogether, whether for convenience or for other reasons such as endometriosis, menstrual migraines, and other discomforts women face while menstruating.

7. News Release. "Many American Women Use Birth Control Pills for Noncontraceptive Reasons." Guttmacher Institute. http://www.guttmacher.org/media/nr/2011/11/15/

Because some of the new continuous birth control and menstrual suppressing methods are fairly new on the market, not enough time has passed for the scientific community to even examine the long-term effects these methods have on women. I will say, however, that suppressing your menstrual cycle and the "normal" shedding of the uterine lining goes against the normal function of the body, and many theorize that this may set up a woman for hormonal issues and/or diseases in her future. Many women will disagree and say the benefits outweigh the risks, but God did design our bodies to menstruate monthly, and interfering with that physiological mechanism is against the natural laws of the body.

Think about it. Birth control is made of synthetic hormones that we put into our body to artificially change our chemical and hormonal structure and to "take control" of those things that are supposed to happen naturally in our bodies. My friend Charity practiced abstinence until she got married, and she felt she was honoring God and herself with this decision. Two weeks into her marriage, however, she was pregnant with her first child. Even though she knew that God is in control and He had blessed her and her husband with their first son, she became angry at her circumstances. Why did it have to happen so soon? She wanted to enjoy her marriage for a little while, not immediately get pregnant and start a family. So, six weeks after having her first son, Charity decided to ban God from the situation and "take control" on her own. She went to her doctor to get the hormonal intrauterine device Mirena. Right away, her husband experienced sharp, needle-like pain from the strings of the IUD during intercourse, so three weeks later she went back to her doctor to trim the strings and all was well. Two and a half years later, she and her husband wanted another child, so the IUD was taken out and she got pregnant two months later.

After the birth of her second child, Charity went again to her doctor to have her IUD inserted. This time, though, things didn't go as planned. After the second insertion of the Mirena device, it punctured her uterus and migrated outside her uterus. At her one-month follow-up appointment, she was given a vaginal exam and an ultrasound, but neither her doctor nor her ultrasound technician was able to find the IUD. She was then sent to the hospital to obtain an X-ray, where they discovered the IUD lodged in front of her colon. She was immediately scheduled for laparoscopic surgery to remove the IUD. The migration of the Mirena device outside the uterus can cause scar tissue or adhesions, infections, blockages and perforations or other damage to other organs. Migration always requires surgery to remove the IUD and in certain cases even necessitates a hysterectomy, resulting in the woman never being able to become pregnant in the future.[8] Luckily, Charity was able to get pregnant just a month later, despite her "birth control" efforts! Looking back, she states that she suffered with extreme mood swings and abnormal behavior while on the Mirena device; hormonally, she was "out of balance." She now realizes that God's plan will be accomplished whether or not you try to control it. She was just fortunate that nothing

> It sounds good to be in control until we learn about some of the adverse reactions that can and do occur.

8. "Mirena IUD Side Effects & Mirena Lawsuits." Lieff Cabraser. http://www.lieffcabraser.com/Personal-Injury/Drugs/Mirena.shtml

more detrimental occurred when her IUD migrated outside her uterus.

Another friend of ours suffered with two years of problems, stemming from an IUD and the mood disturbances it caused. She was initially diagnosed with depression and subsequently prescribed antidepressants. The antidepressants made her mood swings even worse, so her doctor then prescribed mood stabilizers. The side effects and erratic behavior only continued. She then received the diagnosis of bipolar disorder and was prescribed anti-psychotics. However, once her IUD was removed and she weaned herself off the multiple medications, her normal behavior and disposition returned. Obviously, none of her doctors even suspected the IUD, but she now realizes that she is probably not the only woman to have walked this road.

It sounds good to be in control until we learn about some of the adverse reactions that can and do occur. For example, some possible (and immediate) side effects are decreased libido and sex drive. Recent research at Indiana University found that women using the Pill and other hormonal methods reported feeling generally less sexy than those using non-hormonal protection. They had fewer orgasms and less frequent sex, and found it more difficult to get aroused. This starts to defeat the purpose of taking the Pill to begin with![9] Unfortunately, there's more news about the Pill that is most disturbing, as medical research from the UK has shown that hormone replacement therapy and taking the birth control pill may be related to increases in cervical and breast cancer.[10] At the same time, many medical

9. News Release. "Not your mother's birth control, same troubles." http://www.eurekalert.org/pub_releases/2011-10/iu-nym102811.php

10. "The birth control Pill and cancer." Cancer Research UK. http://www.cancerresearchuk.org/cancer-info/healthyliving/hormones/thepill/the-birth-control-pill-and-cancer

news outlets still state that taking artificial hormones—for as long as you want—is perfectly safe!

Ironically, many people in our society will go out of their way to buy "natural pet food" for their cat or dog, or drive a "green" car, as it is well known that petrochemicals pollute the air and can cause health problems and environmental issues; they will speak out against people smoking or drinking, as these artificial chemicals put into the body are harmful, yet they think nothing of a woman taking synthetic hormones for many years. There are risks and benefits to any health decision. A recent Mayo Clinic article states, "You can take birth control pills as long as you need birth control or until you reach menopause, as long as you're generally healthy and don't smoke."[11] Birth control pills may or may not cause XYZ health issue, but consult your health care provider to discuss potential risks versus benefits. The good news is that there are natural solutions to many of the health issues women encounter. Natural methods for birth control, such as Natural Family Planning, may not on the surface appear to be as easy, but I believe our health and longevity are worth the sacrifices we must make at times.

Dealing with your menstrual cycle every month is never truly convenient or something a woman looks forward to, but we have to respect the natural laws of the body. When it comes to dealing with our menstrual cycle, every woman I know faces the monthly routine of using tampons, sanitary napkins and so forth, but many women are also completely unaware of the toxicity and potential dangers of tampons and feminine hygiene products. Some women have no idea that the majority

11. Gallenberg, Mary. "How long can I safely continue taking birth control pills?" Mayo Clinic. http://www.mayoclinic.org/healthy-living/birth-control/expert-answers/birth-control-pills/faq-20058110

of tampons and maxi pads are made with chemicals like bleach, dioxins, synthetic fibers and petrochemical additives. Women need to be aware of this issue, as the average woman will use 16 thousand or more feminine hygiene products in her lifetime.[12] Even worse, the average conventional sanitary pad contains the equivalent of about four plastic bags, according to Andrea Donsky, founder of naturallysavvy.com.[13] This is highly dangerous, as many of us know the harmful effects of BPA (Bisphenol A) and BPS (Bisphenol S), some of the main chemicals in plastic, and their links to heart disease and cancer. Thankfully there are many natural options, such as organic cotton pads and tampons, which are less toxic and widely available, as well as the menstrual cup.

And all women should be aware of a condition called TSS or Toxic Shock Syndrome—a rare bacterial infection that can lead to a potentially fatal drop in blood pressure and organ damage. Most associate it with the use of tampons, particularly super-absorbent varieties that are left in too long. I remember first reading about it on my tampon box. So when my period showed up unexpectedly at midnight, while I was out of town, I asked two of my girlfriends if either one of them had an overnight pad that I could have. Neither one of them did, but one immediately handed me a tampon and said, "Amanda, just use this tonight." I replied, "I can't do that. That's dangerous. You know, because of Toxic Shock Syndrome." They both just laughed at me and said they keep their tampons in overnight

12. Mercola, Joseph. "Women Beware: Most Feminine Hygiene Products Contain Toxic Ingredients." Mercola. http://articles.mercola.com/sites/articles/archive/2013/05/22/feminine-hygiene-products.aspx

13. Donsky, Andrea. "Conventional Hygiene Products: A Women's Issue with Toxic Implications." Naturally Savvy. http://naturallysavvy.com/care/conventional-feminine-hygiene-products-a-womens-issue-with-toxic-implications

all the time. So I just thanked them for the tampon, headed to the concierge, and received some free sanitary napkins from the nice lady behind the front desk.

The internal environment of the vagina, combined with the chemicals found in tampons and a compromised immune system, will allow abnormal amounts of *Staphylococcus aureus* bacteria to live and flourish in some women. Dr. Joseph Mercola of mercola.com suggests the following precautions be taken:

- Avoid super absorbent tampons. Choose the lowest absorbency rate to handle your flow.
- Alternate the use of tampons with sanitary napkins or mini-pads during your period.
- Never leave a tampon inserted overnight; use overnight pads instead.
- Change tampons at least every 4 to 6 hours.
- When inserting a tampon, be extremely careful not to scratch your vaginal lining (avoid plastic applicators).
- Do not use a tampon between periods and also switch to a brand of natural tampons and pads.[14]

Many of these changes may seem challenging at first, but with increased knowledge comes added value and reason for the effort to move in a more natural direction. The Bible states in 1 Corinthians 10:31, "So whether you eat or drink, or whatever you do, do it all for the glory of God." I challenge you all to take one step at a time and make incremental changes for your long-term health.

---

14. Mercola, Joseph. "Dangers of Feminine Hygiene Products that Every Woman Needs to Know." http://articles.mercola.com/sites/articles/archive/2012/01/23/dangers-of-feminine-hygiene-products-every-woman-should-know.aspx

Marianne Mongrello

I grew up in a large, loud, overweight Italian family. Eating, well, *overeating* is what we did best. My weight was always up and down, increasing and decreasing depending on if I was dieting or eating whatever I wanted. My family also excelled at worrying. One of my mother's most famous sayings is, "If you don't worry, it means you don't care!" Most of the aunts and uncles on both sides of my family died from heart disease in their fifties and sixties. Both my brothers and my mom have heart problems; one of my brothers had open heart surgery at age 59.

I was 21 years old when I moved to Atlanta from Boston, and I considered myself to be in very good health. I didn't think about the fact that every summer from the time I was a young teenager, I had strep and spent two weeks in bed. I actually used this yearly malady as a "weight loss" program. The yearly strep throats finally eased up when I was about 25.

At 28, I gave birth to my son, Nick. I have no idea how he was birthed, since they gave me something called "twilight sleep." and when I roused, there he was. I attempted to nurse for about three months, but had a difficult time and no support system, so I began feeding Nick formula. He immediately had terrible colic, vomiting virtually every time he was fed. It was then that he also began having ear infections, and several different strengths of antibiotics did not help, so the pediatrician said the next step would be ear tubes. I had never heard of this, but I was absolutely at a loss as to what to do. I had no one to advise me; my whole family was up north, and I would not go to my husband's family for any kind of advice.

At the same time, my husband began suffering from severe low back pain. He had found a chiropractor in our town who offered to check Nick for us. He then suggested that we let him adjust Nick. Something told me to say yes, though I had never been to a chiropractor or had any idea what they did! For a week, Dr. Preston Cutler came to our home and adjusted my tiny son on his changing table. By the end of that week, his ear infections were gone. We stopped seeing a pediatrician, choosing instead to stay under chiropractic care. I took Nick to Dr. Cutler on a regular basis, but for myself, I went only when my lower back bothered me. As the years went by, I slacked off, but Nick stayed under regular care right up through his mid-teens. He did not see a medical doctor again until he was 15 years old.

On my son's birthday in 2008, I was taken by ambulance to the hospital with stroke level blood pressure. I had been under severe stress for a number of years, but I had no clue that I had blood pressure issues. I was having dizzy spells, and the girls I worked with told me to go to the fire department and have my blood pressure checked. The ENT was the one who took my car keys from me and put me in the ambulance. My blood pressure was 197/114. Four hours later, when I was discharged, my blood pressure was the same. I was told to follow up with a medical doctor, and I did the following week. This began a year of multiple medications, first just two, then two more... and when those did not stabilize my blood pressure, some were replaced with others and even more were added. I wound up at a free clinic due to the loss of my business and my job. The doctors there continued changing, replacing and adding drugs, and I was diagnosed with congestive heart failure.

During this health crisis, I decided to make some lifestyle changes. I switched to unrefined Himalayan salt, I began cardio-exercising and I dramatically increased my water intake. Even with these lifestyle changes and my multitude of blood pressure medications, it was depressing and frightening that my blood pressure continued to be all over the place—not regulated at all.

I had been friends with Jeremy and Amanda Hess for a number of years. I had an interior design business, and they were clients of mine. I started under very sporadic chiropractic care with the Hesses in the early 2000s. In October of 2009, I walked into their office in tears, at the end of my rope, broke, depressed and for the first time in my life, feeling without any hope. They began taking care of me and ultimately changed my life. While taking the blood pressure medications, I had suffered with dizziness, depression, and severe leg aches with walking, as well as a constant dry cough (a known side effect). Within four months of beginning regular chiropractic adjustments along with my lifestyle changes, I weaned off all medication. A year later, my blood pressure stayed at levels normal for my age. Moreover, I no longer had severe sciatic issues.

Four years later, still under chiropractic care, having said goodbye to my Italian eating lifestyle, and drinking lots of water, I am happy to say that my blood pressure gets better with every passing year, and there is no congestive heart failure.

I am in my sixties now, getting senior discounts and Medicare in my near future, and I'm in the minority of the minority of senior citizens and women who are not on any pharmaceuticals. When I analyze my family dynamic, both my brothers and my mom are on blood pressure medication, not to mention a list of other pharmaceuticals as well. One brother has had surgery; one hasn't yet. And my mom has been in and out of the hospital with congestive heart failure. My advice to everyone, and specifically women, is to take better care of yourself in your thirties and forties. Be wise toward your sixties, and create lifestyle habits now to prevent a health crisis in the future.

8.

Just Like Mom

Last week, Jeremy and I were in a friendly argument over some family pictures and which ones were the best to have framed. He sat there looking at me with this grin on his face, when all of a sudden he declared, "You sound just like your mother," then proceeding to snicker at me! At first I denied it wholeheartedly, recalling the Dr. Seuss book I had just read to the kids: "Today you are You, that is truer than true. There is no one alive who is Youer than You..." But later, I thought about what my husband said, and I believe that many of us do sound and/or act like our mothers—which probably isn't such a bad thing, as our mothers carry much wisdom gained from years of life experience, which they then pass on to the next generation. Truth be told, I love it when my daughter Alyssa stands a certain way or gives me these facial expressions that remind me of myself. Maybe Jeremy was somewhat right, after all!

When it comes to health, many women could catch themselves saying something like, "I feel just like my mother," or, "I've got the same problems as my mother," or, "I'm ending up with XYZ condition, just like Mom." If you watch the news, read current health magazines, do web searches on the subject or just simply listen to people in your social circles, you are sure to hear all about how someone's health problem runs in the family… it's "genetic." If we're not careful, we could even take on a victimized identity when referring to our own health problems or concerns, claiming that we didn't have much choice in the matter, as it was predetermined because of our genes. Most of us have heard that current and past research points to the basis of genes or family history as the predetermining factor for our health; however, scientists have been discovering recently that we ourselves play a big part in how our genetic potential expresses itself in terms of our overall health and longevity.

So, if your genetic history is pointing to a certain disease or potential outcome, you can still take steps to decrease the chances of that genetic outcome and shift to a more favorable health outcome.

Research in the field of epigenetics points to the genetic potential that we all have. What we do, how we think, what we put in and on our bodies, our lifestyle habits, etc. all play a role in how our genetic heritage is expressed. So, if your genetic history is pointing to a certain disease or potential outcome, you can still take steps to decrease the chances of that genetic outcome and shift to a more favorable health outcome. *Epigenetics* is the study of changes in organisms caused by modification of gene expression rather than alteration of the genetic code itself. It is the study of gene expression, thus the prefix *epi-* meaning "outside of" or "around" genetics.[1] These changes in gene

1. "Epigenetics." Wikipedia. http://en.wikipedia.org/wiki/Epigenetics

activity may stay for the remainder of the cell's life and may also last for many generations of cells; however, there is no change in the underlying DNA sequence of the organism.[2] Instead, non-hereditary factors cause the organism's genes to behave (express themselves) differently.[3]

The study of epigenetics encourages us to question the common belief held by many of those in the health sciences that your health (or lack thereof) depends on your genetic code, and you are powerless against it. Thankfully, recent studies are showing that although you can't change your DNA or genetic makeup, you can do things to change how it expresses itself in you and your offspring.[4] Cellular biologist Bruce Lipton, PhD. reveals that the cell membrane covering the DNA helps read the DNA inside the cell. The cell membrane receptors pick up "environmental signals" and can choose to read or not to read the genetic code inside that cell. So even if you have the genetic code for cancer "programmed," that doesn't necessarily mean it has to be expressed. The expression is related to environmental (epigenetic) factors, such as emotions, toxins, diet and other choices that affect your mind and body.

You are what you eat.

"You are what you eat." We've all heard this expression, and it's especially true when it comes to pregnancy; your baby is what you eat. Research suggests that pregnant mothers with poor nutrition habits will genetically prime their babies for a

2. Mercola, Joseph. "Falling for This Myth Could Give You Cancer." Mercola. http://articles.mercola.com/sites/articles/archive/2012/04/11/epigenetic-vs-determinism.aspx

3. Mercola, Joseph. "Poor Nutrition in the Womb Triggers Permanent Genetic Changes." Mercola. http://articles.mercola.com/sites/articles/archive/2009/04/30/Poor-Nutrition-in-the-Womb-Triggers-Permanent-Genetic-Changes.aspx

4. Mercola, Joseph. "Falling for This Myth Could Give You Cancer."

nutrient deficient environment. This sets their children up for low birth weights, poor nutrition and a host of diseases like obesity, diabetes and mental and developmental issues. Most interestingly, these studies indicate that the underlying genetic ramifications of poor nutrition possibly can last for two generations, meaning that what your grandmother ate during her pregnancy could be affecting you and your health. Thankfully, epigenetics works in the positive direction too, so making good health choices like whole food and organically based nutrition, supplements, natural cosmetic and homecare products, and chiropractic care while pregnant will move you towards not only the best birth experience possible, but positively shift the health of the next generation! My husband and I hope that this brief discussion of epigenetics will cause people to question a mentality that says, *I have high blood pressure because everyone in my family has it*, or, *I have breast cancer because my mother and grandmother both had it.*

Upon understanding the fundamentals of epigenetics and how much we can do to shift our own genetic outcome, as women we can't ignore the basic health and medical protocols that are deemed necessary to maintain good hygiene and health. I'd like to unwrap two of the more widely recommended ongoing medical tests for women: Pap tests and mammograms. A recent WebMD article states that the second and third most important life-saving tests for women are Pap tests and mammograms (the first is getting checked for heart disease,

> We must prioritize and place value on things and products that will move us in the direction of health for years to come.

and the fourth and fifth are colonoscopy and an annual skin exam, respectively). The article doesn't much discuss prevention, lifestyle habits or epigenetic factors; it suggests to just get the test and if necessary, you will need treatment.[5]

Recently, I went in for my annual checkup, which I don't think any woman looks forward to doing. You take your clothes off in a cold examination room, put on a gown (open in the front) and then put your feet in stirrups while your doctor touches your breast tissue, administers a pelvic exam, and then does a Pap test. During my most recent visit, I decided that I was going to be non-compliant and decline the Pap test. The nurse was taken by surprise as she fumbled her papers and went to speak with the doctor about my request. Then my OBGYN entered the room, asking me the usual questions about my menstrual cycle and any concerns that I may be having. He did his examination and then casually brought up the Pap test. I said, "Doc, I know I'm probably the only woman here declining this today, but I promise to do it next time. Is that okay?"

To my surprise, he responded, "For a healthy, low-risk woman like yourself, that's perfectly fine, and you are getting towards 40, so if everything stays normal you can just do it every couple of years, according to the new guidelines set by the American College of Gynecologists (ACOG)." Growing up thinking that I needed to have this type of testing done annually and then discovering that I didn't need it in the first place left me confused, so when I got home I read the "current" guidelines:

---

5. Mann, Denise. "5 Lifesaving Tests for Women." WebMD. http://www.webmd.com/women/features/5-lifesaving-tests-for-women

Guidelines for Pap Smears

Pap tests should begin at age 21.

From 21-29, it is fine to get a Pap every three years with a cytology screen and no HPV testing.

From 30-65, every three years is acceptable for a Pap test alone (without HPV co-testing) if HPV testing is not available.

From 30-65, co-testing with both cytology and HPV testing is the preferred method every 5 years.

After age 65, you can take Pap smears off your "to-do" list as long as you have had an adequate screening history.

Fryhofer Adamson, Sandra, MD. "The ACOG Cervical Screening Guidelines: Key Changes." http://www.medscape.com/viewarticle/804592

American Cancer Society (ACS), American Society for Colposcopy and Cervical Pathology (ASCCP), and American Society for Clinical Pathology (ASCP). "Cervical Cancer Screening Guidelines for Average-Risk Women." http://www.cdc.gov/cancer/cervical/pdf/guidelines.pdf

The American Congress of Obstetricians and Gynecologists (ACOG). "Ob-Gyns Recommend Women Wait 3 to 5 Years Between Pap Tests." http://www.acog.org/About-ACOG/News-Room/News-Releases/2012/Ob-Gyns-Recommend-Women-Wait-3-to-5-Years-Between-Pap-Tests

After reading the current guidelines, I wondered how many women every day get this questionably unnecessary type of testing, not knowing that ACOG has changed its guidelines. Then I thought to myself, *Is it totally necessary for me to get an annual pelvic exam?* To my delight, new guidelines published in the Annals of Internal Medicine recommend that healthy, low-risk women not have routine annual pelvic exams.[6] The panel of experts found no benefit from the annual pelvic exam except that it caused women discomfort, distress, and sometimes, even unnecessary surgeries. ACOG, however, still recommends a yearly pelvic exam for women, even though it acknowledges that the evidence does not support or refute its value for a low-risk patient with no symptoms.[7]

To conclude my story at the OBGYN, as he told me that I could spread out my Pap smears, in the next breath he reminded me that since I would be 40 in the near future I would need to start my mammograms. I replied, "Thanks, and have a great day," relieved that he was so pleasant and accommodating toward me. Then, I started to contemplate annual mammograms. The whole concept of mammograms always has bothered me, and while I understand that the medical community touts this test as a life-saving diagnostic tool, I have always thought to myself that mammography is radiation… and radiation causes cancer…so why would you want to radiate your breast tissue intentionally year after year? Thus the topic of mammograms is another subject of scrutiny in the natural health community.

6. LeWine, Howard. "Expert panel says healthy women don't need yearly pelvic exam." Harvard Health Blog. http://www.health.harvard.edu/blog/expert-panel-says-healthy-women-dont-need-yearly-pelvic-exam-201407027250

7. News Release. "ACOG Practice Advisory on Annual Pelvic Examination Recommendations." ACOG. http://www.acog.org/About-ACOG/News-Room/College-Statements-and-Advisories/2014/ACOG-Practice-Advisory-on-Annual-Pelvic-Examination-Recommendations

At the start of my research, I was shocked when I read a *Huffington Post* article that explains the founding of National Breast Cancer Awareness Month (NBCAM) by the American Cancer Society (ACS), the world's largest nonprofit organization. The NBCAM was founded in 1984, with National Mammography Day as its flagship event. The NBCAM, which takes place every October, was conceived and funded by the Imperial Chemical Industries, a leading international manufacturer of petrochemicals, and its US subsidiary Zeneca Pharmaceuticals. Zeneca is the sole manufacturer of Tamoxifen, which has been widely used for treating breast cancer.[8] And while the ACS still claims that early detection via mammography has a close to 100 percent cure rate, they fail to report that one mammogram emits an amount of radiation equivalent to 1,000 chest X-rays! Dr. Samuel Epstein, Chairman of the Cancer Prevention Coalition, has stated:

> The premenopausal breast is highly sensitive to radiation, each 1 rad exposure increasing breast cancer risk by about 1 percent, with a cumulative 10 percent increased risk for each breast over a decade's screening.[9]

That leaves the question of risk versus benefit when discussing the controversial topic of mammography. The most recent mammogram guidelines from the US Preventive Services Task Force recommend "most" women begin screening at

8. Epstein, Samuel. "Breast Cancer Unawareness Month: Rethinking Mammograms." Huffington Post. http://www.huffingtonpost.com/samuel-s-epstein/the-breast-cancer-unaware_b_754641.html

9. Mercola, Joseph. "Your Greatest Weapon Against Breast Cancer (Not Mammograms)." Mercola. http://articles.mercola.com/sites/articles/archive/2012/03/03/experts-say-avoid-mammograms.aspx

age 50 and repeat the test every two years through the age of 74. These guidelines; however, have not been accepted by the ACS or ACOG, who still tout age 40 as the time to begin mammograms.[10] This would explain my OBGYN's comment, since he would have to adhere to the guidelines set by ACOG. As it turns out, the ACS has financial ties to the mammography industry, so it would financially make sense for them to keep recommending mammograms to women starting at an earlier age.[11]

An alternative though controversial diagnostic tool for breast screening is *high-definition thermal imaging*, or *thermography*. It checks and detects heat differentials of the body, or the part of the body under evaluation, and generates information that can help with a diagnosis or treatment options. Best of all, thermal imaging is non-invasive, as the scanner just glides over the surface of the body, and it is totally painless; also, unlike a mammogram, it is not an X-ray, so no ionizing radiation is involved. What's the downside, then? Since the medical community has been invested for such a long time in mammography, they are very slow to come around to recognize thermography; because of that, in most cases health insurance will not cover thermal imaging. Unfortunately, the medical community states that there is very little scientific evidence or studies to support the use of thermal imaging in the early detection of breast cancer in women who are *asymptomatic*, meaning they do not have symptoms. Additionally, there are

10. Pruthi, Sandhya. "With differing mammogram guidelines, I'm not sure when to begin mammogram screening. What does Mayo Clinic recommend?" Mayo Clinic. http://www.mayoclinic.org/tests-procedures/mammogram/expert-answers/mammogram-guidelines/faq-20057759

11. Mercola, Joseph. "Mammogram: The Cancer Test That's a Death Trap..." Mercola. http://articles.mercola.com/sites/articles/archive/2010/09/02/cancer-society-has-financial-ties-to-mammography.aspx

no scientific studies comparing the effectiveness of thermal imaging versus mammography in asymptomatic women.

Samuel S. Epstein, MD, who has written multiple books on the cancer industry, has stated (along with others in the health field) that many organizations, including the American Cancer Society, fall short on the conversation surrounding lifestyle changes and limiting the risks of breast cancer and cancer in general, as much is now known about cancer.[12] What are some measures that you can take to counteract cancer or just be healthier, feel great and extend your longevity? I always say that you can't control the number of years you will be around—only God controls that—but I believe you and I have much to do with the quality of life of the years God grants us. We really need to make the most of them, for our family's sake and for the purpose God has for us. For specifics, Dr. Jeremy and I cover our List of Healthy Living To-Dos in the last chapter of the book.

I find that it's all too common in society that in so many cases, when a life-threatening disease such as breast or cervical cancer is presented, an analysis of lifestyle habits is rarely a consideration. I'm not claiming that if you attain to a healthy, organic diet and moderate exercise, your structure and nervous system are in balance with chiropractic, and you utilize as many natural living approaches possible, you won't ever get sick. However, just like taking care of your teeth, if you brush and floss, you greatly reduce your chances of dental cavities or gum disease, the same goes for the majority of health concerns and

12. Mercola, Joseph. "Your Greatest Weapon Against Breast Cancer (Not Mammograms)." Mercola. http://articles.mercola.com/sites/articles/archive/2012/03/03/experts-say-avoid-mammograms. aspx

diseases of the body. I believe that God created our bodies with an innate intelligence, which knows exactly what our bodies need at all times to function properly and to be whole, and when we do what is best for our bodies, then we increase the likelihood of our bodies ability to heal themselves and avoid disease. Not one person is perfect (not even me), but while making daily, consistent decisions for your health potential and longevity definitely is not easy, it is a must. We should respect and honor the "temple" that God has given us on our journey to live out our soul purpose for Him. I believe so many people won't and don't reach the potential God has put in them, simply because their health suffers so much.

Everyone, including myself, comes into contact with various epigenetic factors knowingly or unknowingly, but we all can make choices on a daily basis of where we spend our time, energy and money. We must prioritize and place value on things and products that will move us in the direction of health for years to come. It never ceases to amaze me how some people will tell me they have no time to exercise, whether at the gym or at home, but then I catch them trying to tell me about their favorite TV show. Or they say they can't afford buying organic food, but they always have the latest technology gadgets. The point is that in many cases, it is not a lack of money, but a lack of value. Sometimes this lack of value comes from a lack of knowledge. The media won't inform you, your doctor in most cases is just following protocols, and your friends, sisters and mothers are most likely uninformed themselves. You and I don't have to be the victims of ignorance. Every woman should find her own path and follow her own truth and decisions. Get informed, take responsibility for your health, and feel good about your choices.

> *For we must all stand before Christ to be judged*
> *and have our lives laid bare—before Him.*
> *Each of us will receive whatever he deserves*
> *for the good or bad things he has done in his earthly body.*
> —2 Corinthians 5:10, *Living Bible (TLB)*

Waist Line

Dr. Amanda Hess

"Amanda, look at yourself in the mirror. Suck your stomach in! Stand up straight! Tuck your butt in and pull up! You look fat." I was nine years old, wearing a black leotard and pink tights, with my hair pulled up in a bun. When my ballet instructor said those demoralizing words to me in front of the whole class, I wanted to cry, but I did as she said because I wanted to be the next great ballerina dancing on my tiptoes onstage, with the audience giving me a standing ovation.

Although this was the first time that I was ever deemed "fat," it only bothered me for a brief second. I grew up feeling very awkward about myself with friends of mine always saying how skinny I was. I was the girl who could eat anything and everything. When I was in middle school I became an apprentice at the local ballet company where we had "weigh-ins" every so often. It never bothered me because I was the underweight, bony type, but even at that young age I remember some of the more developed, heavier girls getting reprimanded for their weight. In high school, I was not the athlete on the sports team. I was the lightweight "flyer" on top of the cheerleading pyramid for 2 years, until a major fall made me disenchanted with cheering because it had affected my dancing capabilities. The funny thing now about the fall was that it led me to my local chiropractor for the first time.

I was so skinny that I envied all the other girls who were developing faster than I was. The local neighborhood boys even made fun of me during the summertime because I was this tall, skinny girl who couldn't fill out a bikini whatsoever. It was so mortifying. But dancing gave me an escape—a way to express myself. I got to dress up in amazing costumes with my hair and makeup done, which made me feel beautiful. So, in high school I continued dancing, dancing, and dancing. I even skipped my junior prom because of a dance performance. In high school, the administration allowed us to go off-campus for lunch, so my friends and I ate at places like Subway, Taco Bell, Wendy's, and my favorite, Bojangles'. At Subway, I would eat a 6-inch turkey sub, a bag of chips, a chocolate chip cookie, and get a soft drink. A typical week for me also included 1-2 boxes of Little Debbie Fudge Rounds—my all-time favorite snack growing up. At Bojangles', the best fried chicken in the South (my opinion only), my meal was always the fried chicken breast dinner with seasoned fries, a butter biscuit and sweet South Carolina tea. I think the only reason I stayed so skinny is because I was burning so many calories dancing everyday. I graduated high school second in my class at about 120 pounds and wearing a size 6.

In 1994, I entered the University of South Carolina to obtain a degree in biology. I joined a sorority and began a college life of parties, tailgating and eating late at night, with some studying mixed in here and there. I continued to exercise at a local gym, but not to the degree that I had been when dancing. The late nights, parties and my poor eating habits evenutally caught up to me. I gained a tremendous amount of weight, going from a size 6 to a size 10. Since I was so tall, it didn't really bother me until my second year of college. I had moved onto the sorority floor with all the other beautiful girls. My roommate that year was a girl that I didn't really know until we became roomies. Her name was Susan. She happened to be good friends with some of the other girls already.

During the course of that year, I was introduced to the concept of eating disorders. I had heard about them, but never really knew anyone with one. Come to find out, my neighbor next to us was anorexic, the girl down the hall was also anorexic, and it seemed everybody was on a diet and taking diet pills. And then, I had the pleasure of watching Susan waste away, going to a low weight of about 85 pounds. Her parents attempted to intervene and let her finish out the school year, but I will never forget living with her and watching her eat a bag of grapes for dinner, or worse yet, microwaving Green Giant Brussels sprouts and spraying I Can't Believe It's Not Butter on them as her meal for the day—all while she carefully cut them in half perfectly and ate them ever so slowly. With my roommate wasting away and other sorority members starving themselves too made for quite a life-altering experience. The problem for me was that I loved food too much to starve myself. So I just began going to the gym not once per day but twice per day. Before classes I would hit the gym at 5 AM, and then I would go again around 7 PM. I would also go through periods of "dieting," and I would lose 5 to 10 pounds, but with my party lifestyle and poor eating habits, the pounds always came back on.

The following year, Susan's parents kept her home in Virginia and she never returned to South Carolina. I attempted to call her a few times, but she never responded, so I gave up. I skipped some sorority meetings and functions because my academics needed more attention. I got reprimanded for my absence while other girls were failing their classes, so I decided to quit the sorority and move off-campus with an old friend of mine from high school. She was working at the mall as a store manager and I was still in school, also working part-time at the local hospital. I continued to exercise like crazy but never really understood how to eat properly. My new roommate was my longtime friend from high school, Kim. She was a pretty, petite, and ever-so-skinny Asian girl with perfect, flowing black hair. While living with her, I noticed that she too never really ate a lot. Many days it appeared she would eat only one meal per day.

I also began hanging out with another college friend of mine, Jennifer who also was skinny, but she seemed to eat rather healthy. It wasn't until one late night after partying that my life changed. Jennifer and I were heading home when we stopped at a 24-hour diner for a snack. We had done this many times before, but this time for whatever reason she said she had to go to the bathroom and I went with her. Instead of going to the bathroom, I watched her proceed to vomit up her food. I was speechless. I asked her about it, and she basically said that sometimes she threw up her food and that helped her stay thin. The concept of it just grossed me out. Then one day after being fed up with exercising all the time and not being able to slim down, I decided, why not. It seemed everyone else was doing it; it must not be that big of a deal. So I ate whatever I wanted (remember I loved food so much that I wasn't going to starve myself) and then I stuck my finger down my throat and vomited all of it into the toilet. This was the start of the most painful part of my young adult life. And yes, I did lose a tremendous amount of weight but then I lost all sense of how to eat normally and feared gaining any weight again. I loved the way I looked, but I was destroying my body. I achieved a low of 115 pounds, which included 2 hospitalizations and countless therapy sessions. One medical doctor told me that Prozac would cure me. I believed him. What a joke! The only thing Prozac did for me was provide me with more erratic behavior, hallucinations, and suicidal thoughts.

Even though I had no relationship with God at the time and I grew up going to church mainly just on Easter and Christmas, I clearly remember being in my bathroom after another episode, crying out to God that if He were real, then He would save me. That I knew that I couldn't break free of my addiction by myself. It had already taken over. I asked Jesus to help me, but I had still never accepted Him as my Lord and Savior.

Fast forward to meeting my husband, Jeremy, who for whatever reason believed in me, attended countless nutritional sessions with me, and taught me how to eat more naturally and healthy. With his support and us attending a local church on an "irregular" basis, I finally turned my life over to God, accepted Jesus Christ as my Savior and asked for forgiveness and healing. Once I did that, food became less of my focus. That same year, I stopped my eating disorder completely and began to take responsibility for myself. I believe that more people are addicted to food than even pharmaceutical or street drugs, pornography, gambling, smoking, alcohol, etc. Whether they are starving themselves or overeating, many people never truly conquer their food demons. And with our food supply so tainted in today's society, it's no wonder society seems to be getting sicker and sicker. When people ask us about how we eat or our lifestyle habits, we typically don't have time to go into everything, but here is a short list as a starting point:

1. We never eat fast food. The closest we get to eating fast food is at an airport, where we will get a salad from a place like Qdoba.
2. We eat mainly proteins and vegetables, and some fruit.
3. We eat/cook/bake gluten-free pastas, breads and desserts on a very infrequent basis. My weaknesses are still granola and oats. If I eat them in moderation, I seem to function fine. If I overeat these carbohydrates, I feel bloated and my digestive system gets irritated.
4. We never drink soft drinks and we don't have any at the house. We mainly drink water, and some kefir or homemade fruit smoothies for the kids. Our one vice is a good cup of coffee or a latté with almond milk (although almond milk does not froth that well).
5. We buy only organic meat and poultry for the house and attempt to buy as much organic fruits and vegetables as possible. Sometimes, certain fruits and vegetables are only sold conventionally, so we may have to budge in those cases.
6. We don't use synthetic hormonal contraception.
7. We have a full house water filtration system.

8. Our household cleaning products, skincare products, and personal care products are either organic or as natural as we can find.

9. We exercise regularly, but we're not extreme exercise enthusiasts.

We are both in our late 30s (which is hard to believe). I weigh 125-129 pounds, and I usually fit into a size 2 or extra small. So yes, I am thin. I do believe the apparel industry has changed, in that I weighed 5 to 10 pounds less when graduating high school and yet I wore a size 6. I get very bloated when I eat a lot of carbohydrates, e.g. cereal, granola or chips. I still have a sweet tooth, so you will see me eating vegan chocolate chip cookies, yogurt, or a piece of a dark chocolate bar. And I love chai lattés or mochas made with almond milk.

Our menus for a typical day would be:

- **Breakfast**: eggs made scrambled, poached, or fried; a nutritional shake made with berries, water, and stevia; one cup of coffee
- **Lunch**: bison sliders (no bun); vegetable medley of brussel sprouts, carrots, onions, and broccoli
- **Dinner**: ginormous salad with some sort of protein
- Water throughout the day
- **Snacks**: anything from fresh organic fruit; yogurt and granola; guacamole; nuts/trail mix; cut veggies

I am not writing this for people to dissect and either agree and/or disagree with how we eat. It is a fact that anytime you are eating out of a box or at a fast food or chain restaurant, you have to understand that the food is just not as nutritious for you. You can exercise everyday and still not lose the unwanted pounds if you are eating sugar, carbohydrates, fast food, and chemically laden, hormonally enhanced food and beverages.

The biggest obstacle we face today in regards to our "waistlines" is not ourselves anymore, but is in dealing with our children. I would be lying if I said that our children eat as well as we do, but I can say honestly that they eat better than their classmates. It is a daily struggle between my husband and myself trying to get them to eat protein, vegetables, fruit and water versus them wanting cereal, pasta, chips, cookies, sugar-filled juices, etc. When they were each three years old, both of our children filled out a questionnaire about me as a Mother's Day activity with their teacher. Most of the answers were quite comical, but one question was answered perfectly.

My Mommy's favorite food is _____ .
My daughter Alyssa answered *salad*.
My son Gabriel answered *Brussels sprouts.*

I would love to say that my children's favorite foods are salad and Brussels sprouts. Hopefully one day I can, but until then I will continue to fight the fight and teach them to make the best choices possible for their health.

9.
Natural Living: Designed by God

Life happens, the kids grow up fast and the years go by quickly! God granted us our lives to glorify Him. We believe that God gives each of us a purpose, and we also believe that in order to live out that destiny, we've got to nurture, care for and protect our bodies. We make daily choices to improve and optimize our health. Good health is freely given to us when we are born, and taking consistent steps to gain and keep superior health is essential to a life full of purpose, one that fulfills His calling on our lives.

We believe so many people sabotage their purposeful life because they neglect their health, which ultimately causes long-term, negative ramifications. True health resides in the daily decisions, those moments that happen dozens of times a day. It's in simple choices like, *Should I take the elevator or walk the stairs? Do I grab soda or spring water at the convenience store? Do I wake up 30 minutes early to take a walk and exercise or ignore my body's need for movement? Should I cook a nutritious breakfast of eggs and fruit or hit the fast food drive-through, again?* We could go on and on, and we are challenged with the same decisions as everyone else. Analyze your lifestyle and ask yourself if you are making choices that are adding to or subtracting from your health. Are you letting life just happen and placing the blame on your genetics, or are you taking responsibility for your health?

In chiropractic philosophy, we use the terms *constructive survival value* and *destructive survival value*. Things in life that we choose to do, say, think or act upon will cause either constructive or destructive outcomes to our lives—and our health. We set out writing this *Designed by God* series for two reasons: the first, to teach people why they should question and analyze the current healthcare system and their beliefs concerning health; and the second (and more important), to provide a variety of solutions about how each of us can make daily incremental changes to achieve better health. One of our favorite competitive quotes from Tim Duncan is, "Good, better, best. Never let it rest. Until your good is better and your better is best." With this in mind, we thought we would share our top 20 solutions and strategies for healthy living. We practice all these on a regular basis so that we can fulfill God's purpose for our lives, in addition to attaining as much health and longevity possible—not so much for ourselves, but for the people who need us most.

Below are our Top 20 Healthy Living To-Dos, which are solutions and strategies to address problems affecting a large percentage of women, many of whom are unaware and uninformed.

1. **Regular Chiropractic Care**. Okay, so we are biased on this one, but we have to say that we're not only biased, but also right! A regular chiropractic adjustment (for the whole family) is

one of the biggest overall health benefits totally missed by even the most educated natural health consumer. The bottom line is your spine, also known as your vertebral column, is formed from individual bones called vertebrae, which house and protect the spinal cord. If these bones are out of their proper alignment, it results in nerve interference. We always say, "Proper structure equals proper function." Since your nervous system controls the function of the body, doesn't it just make sense to make sure your spinal column is in proper alignment? Simply put, your body functions better without nerve interference.

2. **Organic Food and Beverages.** Did you know that organic fruit and vegetables contain up to 40 percent more antioxidants, organic produce has higher levels of beneficial minerals like iron and zinc, and milk from organic herds contain up to 90 percent more antioxidants?[1] Now, some people reading this will say they can't afford to buy organic; well, for your long-term health, you can't afford *not* to buy organic. Certain conventional (non-organic) food contains more antibiotics, hormones or pesticides than others, so look at what you're buying and maximize your budget accordingly. We believe it is the cumulative effect of these types of chemicals that affects overall health.

3. **Water for Life.** Everyone knows that they should drink a certain amount of water every day. But what type of water? In most cities, normal tap water is chemically treated so that it's safe for consumption, but is it truly safe? There are also many bottled waters (purified waters) that put city water through

1. Paddock, Catharine. "Organic Food Is More Nutritious Say EU Researchers." Medical News Today. http://www.medicalnewstoday.com/articles/86972.php

reverse osmosis to clean the water, but then chemicals are put back into it. If we are traveling, we buy "spring water" not "pure drinking water," as the law now mandates that manufacturers must state the difference on the bottle. When able, we always choose a glass bottle over a plastic one, and if we are close to home, we will fill up one or more glass bottles at the house before we leave and throw them in the car for the kids and ourselves.

4. **Soaps, Suds & Skincare.** Your skin, the largest organ in your body, absorbs everything you put on it. Most people never give a thought as to what chemicals, toxins or dangerous substances may be lurking in the things they rub on themselves or clean their houses with. All kinds of parabens, phthalates, preservatives, alcohol, dyes and colorings are loaded into cosmetics, skincare and household products. The Environmental Working Group's Cosmetic Safety Database (www.ewg.org/skindeep/) is a must for any person wondering or curious about what's in their favorite soap, skincare, sunscreen or toothpaste. Consider swapping all laundry, dishwashing, and household cleaning products for natural, organically based options, which can be found online or at a local natural foods store.

5. **Artificial Sweeteners.** Many of these are marketed under names like Splenda, NutraSweet, Sweet N' Low, Equal, etc. All are artificial in nature and produced in a laboratory. Consider using sugar in the raw, stevia, honey or other natural sweeteners.

6. **Sunscreen.** Did you know that certain chemicals in sunscreens are considered *photocarcinogenic*? This means that when these chemicals are exposed to light, they become a carcinogen (a cancer-causing agent)! Some of the worst offenders are "baby" or "toddler" sunscreens. Study your sunscreens and protect yourself accordingly.

7. **Tampons & Feminine Hygiene.** This is simple: search for organic cotton tampons and maxi pads free of chlorine, dyes and fragrances. Another option is an insertable menstrual cup, which unlike tampons, does not absorb your menstrual flow but collects it. Most menstrual cups do not contain any of the following: latex, plastic, PVC, acrylic, acrylate, BPA, phthalate, elastomer, polyethylene, colors or dyes, which makes them a safer option.

8. **Consider Limiting and/or Eliminating Bread, Pizza & Pasta.** Don't hate on us—we're not saying never to eat these things, but do consider drastically reducing them and their friends—donuts, bagels, pastries, cake, pancakes, toast, etc. When someone asks how we stay so slim and comments that we must be exercising all the time, or that we must be vegetarians, we immediately respond, "Stop eating bread, pizza, pasta and their friends," especially at night. Our family may go out for pizza as a treat once every six to eight weeks; we rarely buy bread at the house, and only then to appease our kids so they can occasionally take an almond butter and jelly sandwich for lunch and feel semi-normal at school; and we limit pasta, choosing brands that are gluten-free and made from brown rice or quinoa.

9. **See a Naturopath.** If you're like us and you know you don't want pharmaceuticals thrown at you when you go to the doctor, then we would recommend getting a good naturopathic doctor to advise and care for you and your family when the need arises. They will care for your health concerns with proper nutrition, supplements and other natural solutions. Check www.naturopathic.org to find a doctor near you.

10. **Keep Your Body Moving.** This seems very elementary, but too many people neglect their skeletal and muscular systems. We fully know and understand that it takes effort to eke out time in a busy schedule to exercise and get moving. If the kids want to ride bikes, we will ride bikes with them or walk/run alongside of them. In the summertime, we play with them in the pool but also will do some lap swimming. We also carve out time when the kids are either asleep or in school, doing yoga or interval training with free weights and cardiovascular equipment. Find out what type of exercise you like to do, and just make time for it.

11. **HFCS, MSG & Friends.** The food industry is notorious for hiding these things in our foods. High fructose corn syrup, monosodium glutamate (MSG), aspartame, preservatives, food colorings, artificial flavors and synthetic trans fats are some of the most dangerous ingredients to look out for. Unfortunately, the food industry has altered the names of these dangerous substances many times, so when you read an ingredients list, you may not even recognize the danger lurking in that particular product! The best policy to adopt immediately is to buy as little

packaged and processed foods as possible. When we go grocery shopping, less than 20 percent of our groceries actually go into the pantry; the rest is all perishable—products like eggs, meats, poultry and a ton of fruits and vegetables. We say when you visit the grocery store, shop the walls, and not the aisles, which contain canned/boxed foods that in many cases have a shelf life of several *years*.

12. **Birth Control and Hormone Replacement Therapy (HRT).** In our opinion, synthetic hormone use is neither natural nor completely safe. Practice abstinence if you are not married, and when you are married, consider natural family planning methods (www.natural-family-planning.info/standard-days-method.htm) Some people also practice barrier methods during times of increased fertility. Talk to your partner and figure out what is best for you.

In regards to HRT, use of hormone-replacement drugs fell sharply after 2002 when the Women's Health Initiative, a major government research trial, found that they raised the risk of heart attack and stroke in older women. Recently, you will find some new studies stating that short-term HRT seems to be safe now for early menopausal women. Consider other herbal and supplemental options first and talk to your naturopath about your choices.

13. **Routine Diagnostic Testing.** Be careful of just jumping into any diagnostic testing your doctor recommends. Over-utilization of many diagnostic tests is far too common. Do your research as current guidelines continue to change.

14. **Fluoride.** We all remember learning about the benefits of fluoride and brushing our teeth with fluoride-containing toothpaste for good dental health. However, we would suggest reading information challenging this doctrine. Our family uses non-fluoride products (against the recommendations of our local dentist) and a house water filtration system to clean our water of a lot of things…including fluoride! Check out www.fluoridealert.org for more information.

15. **Microwave Ovens.** Most never discuss or even think about it, but microwave ovens are downright dangerous! Your food is chemically altered when you use a microwave. Even worse, many people use plastic in the microwave. As the plastic heats up, it leaches chemicals from the plastic into your food. This is yet another controversial topic, and you should research and decide what is best for your family. We haven't had a microwave in our house for over nine years.

16. **Birthing Options.** We believe that women need to get educated on the birthing process. There are many options to having a natural birthing process and a healthy pregnancy. We are so passionate about this that one of the books in the *Designed by God* series is *Baby Designed by God*, which covers healthy pregnancy, natural birth and raising drug-free children.

17. **Connect with a Good Natural Foods Store.** Depending on where you live, this might be a larger store like Whole Foods or Sprouts, but in some urban and rural areas, this might be a natural foods co-op, herb shop or health food store. Whichever it is, get to know the people who work there and don't be afraid

to ask questions or try new items. We love exploring any natural foods market and trying new food when we travel to different places!

18. **Avoid Pharmaceutical Drugs**. This would seem like a no-brainer, but according to the Mayo Clinic, 7 out of 10 Americans are taking one or more drugs on a daily basis![2] 25 percent of women in certain age groups are on anti-depressants, and many are taking statins (cholesterol drugs) even though new studies show they increase the risk of diabetes in women by 48 percent.[3, 4] Remember, God created the body to heal itself and gave it everything it needs; we just need to take care of it.

19. **Reduce Stress**. Stress can be one of the main causes of all types of health problems and concerns. The best way we eliminate stress is through meditation and prayer. Reading and speaking God's Word over our lives and situations, and casting our worries, fears and concerns onto Him is the best stress reliever. We rest knowing that He is our Rock and foundation. You don't need to read the Bible or meditate on it all day—just a bit each day. Another good stress-reducing step is to limit or eliminate watching the news and other TV programming. It would seem that plopping down in front of the TV at the end

2. "Nearly 7 in 10 Americans Take Prescription Durgs, Mayo Clinic, Olmstead Medical Center Find." Mayo Clinic News Network. http://newsnetwork.mayoclinic.org/discussion/nearly-7-in-10-americans-take-prescription-drugs-mayo-clinic-olmsted-medical-center-find

3. Bindley, Katherine. "Women and Perscription Drugs: One in Four Takes Mental Health Meds." *Huffington Post*. http://www.huffingtonpost.com/2011/11/16/women-and-prescription-drug-use_n_1098023.html

4. Hyman, Mark. "Why Women Should Stop Their Cholesterol Lowering Medication." Dr. Mark Hyman. http://drhyman.com/blog/2012/01/19/why-women-should-stop-their-cholesterol-lowering-medication/

of a long day would be relaxing, but the TV keeps your mind moving in stressful patterns, especially when it is the typical negative news broadcast.

20. **Never Stop Learning.** Before taking the indoctrinated advice of a family member, friend, doctor or the media, do your due diligence, research and make *informed* decisions about what you think is best for your health and the health of your family. We always say, "Tell me the health attitudes or perspectives of your 5 closest friends, and that will be a large determining factor in your personal health future."

We hope this book and the *Designed by God* series has given you clarity on many health topics and solutions related to women and their families. We believe that we are accomplishing our mission, one that inspires people to live and move in a direction of natural living, to find freedom in knowing God gave our bodies everything they need, an amazing ability to heal themselves and the promise of good health and longevity. We would love to hear your story, too. Reach out to us at DrsHess@ Designed-by-God.com and join the Facebook group "Natural Living Designed by God." Go online and visit our resource guides on Designed-by-God.com. If you are reading this book, you know women we don't know, and with knowledge comes responsibility. Please share our message of hope and healing with women in your life!

Moving the World toward Natural Health,
Drs. Amanda & Jeremy Hess

ABOUT THE AUTHORS

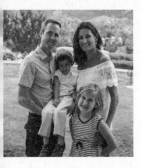

Dr. Jeremy Hess is a practicing chiropractor in Georgia since 2000. He is a graduate of Life University, a member of the Georgia Council of Chiropractic since 1998, a board member since 2007, and serving as Vice President from 2010-2013. He is a member of the International Chiropractic Pediatric Association, National Vaccine Information Center, International Federation of Chiropractors & Organizations and a Lifetime Member of the International Chiropractors Association.

Dr. Amanda Hess is a practicing chiropractor in the state of Georgia since 2003. She completed college as a graduate of the University of South Carolina with a Bachelor's of Science degree in Biology and her Doctorate of Chiropractic degree at Life University. She is a member of the Georgia Council of Chiropractic, League of Chiropractic Women, International Chiropractic Pediatric Association, National Vaccine Information Center, International Federation of Chiropractors & Organizations and a lifetime member of the International Chiropractors Association.

Drs. Jeremy and Amanda Hess own and operate the busiest chiropractic practice in Stockbridge Ga., the busiest in the state and one of the busiest in the world. They also mentor and teach chiropractors and students practice procedures and inspire them to make a huge impact in their communities thru their "AMPED" Mentorship and Development program for chiropractors and natural health providers.

They live in Lake Spivey, GA with their two children, Alyssa and Gabriel. Their mission is to serve God by serving the families of his community and region through principled chiropractic care allowing the Innate healing potential of the body to fully express itself.

THE DESIGNED BY GOD SERIES

Live a Natural, Holistic Life Based on God's Design

Join the Community, Share Your Story and
Find Resources to Live a Heathy Life.

www.designed-by-god.com

www.facebook.com/Designedbygodbook

www.twitter.com/DBGBook

www.google.com/+Designed-by-god

The first book in the series:

BABY designed by God

After impacting thousands of readers,
Amazon bestseller *Baby Designed by God*
continues to enlighten mothers and fathers
from all backgrounds.

**AVAILABLE WHEREVER
FINE BOOKS ARE SOLD**

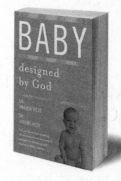